— Healthy Cooking —

HIGH FIBRE
COOKBOOK

Healthy Cooking

HIGH FIBRE
COOKBOOK

Paul Morgan

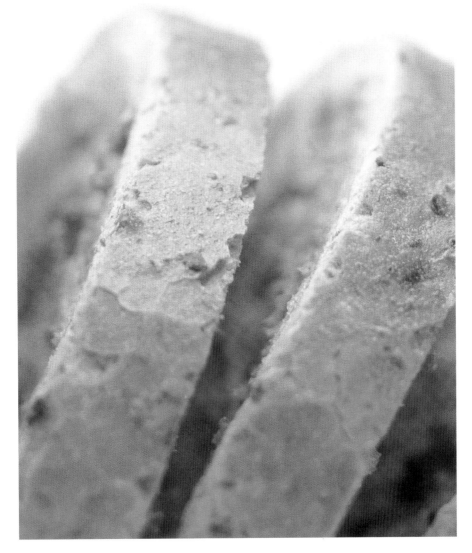

AN OCEANA BOOK

This edition published by Silverdale Books,
an imprint of Bookmart Ltd., in 2006

Bookmart Ltd.
Blaby Road
Wigston
Leicester
LE18 4SE

ISBN 1-84509-234-1

QUMHCHF

Manufactured in Singapore by
Pica Digital Pte. Ltd.
Printed in Singapore by
Star Standard Industries (Pte) Ltd

It is always sensible to consult your doctor before changing your diet
regime, but it is essential to do so if you suffer from any medical
condition or are taking medication of any kind. If you are concerned about
any symptoms that develop after changing your diet, consult your doctor
immediately. Information is given without any guarantees on the part of the
author and publisher, and they cannot be held responsible for the
contents of this book.

CONTENTS

INTRODUCTION

Scientists have known for a long time that a diet rich in fibre is good for you, but many people still do not know just how good it is. It is true that the publication in 1982 of the hugely successful The F-Plan Diet drew the public's attention to a high-fibre, low-fat diet's potential as part of a weight-loss regime, but many people still do not realize how vitally important fibre is to their health. Though fibre may play an essential part in a healthy diet, just what – since this is a healthy eating cookbook – is a healthy diet?

For 25 years or more, theories about what constitutes a healthy diet have chopped and changed. Take your heart and circulatory system, for example. First, all fat was considered to be bad for you – then it was found that some types of fat can protect your heart. Then butter was considered bad, while margarine was thought to be good for you – but after a while, scientists discovered that margarine contained substances called trans fatty acids, which are extremely bad for you. At the same time, all cholesterol was once considered dangerous, but now we know that one type of cholesterol is, in fact, very good for you.

And for 17 of these 25 years, scientists tended to mock the insistent claims made by practitioners of fringe and alternative medicine to the effect that people could prevent cancer from developing if they ate the correct diet. But in 1997, the doubters were proved wrong, when the World Cancer Research Fund and the American Institute for Cancer Research (AIRC) published a joint study that was the culmination of 15 years of research. In it, they stated

'The panel found that . . . inappropriate diets cause around one-third of all cancer deaths . . . . [it] estimates that 30 to 40 per cent of cancer cases throughout the world are preventable by feasible dietary means'.

You could be forgiven for being confused. But now, after years of research, scientists have a fairly clear picture of the relationship between nutrition and disease. The basic facts are now known: it is beyond question that by eating a healthy diet and avoiding some foods while emphasizing others you can not only lose weight but significantly reduce your chances of developing diseases of the heart and arteries and contracting many types of cancer. And a healthy diet emphasizes the amount of fibre and reduces the amount of fat that you eat.

This book will show you how to eat healthily and lose weight. First we will look at what fibre is and how it affects your body. Then we will show how the make-up of some foods can cause disease while the chemical basis of other foods can prevent it. Then you can choose from a range of mouth-watering, high-fibre, healthy recipes. It may be a cliché, but like many clichés it is true: when it comes to your health, you really are what you eat!

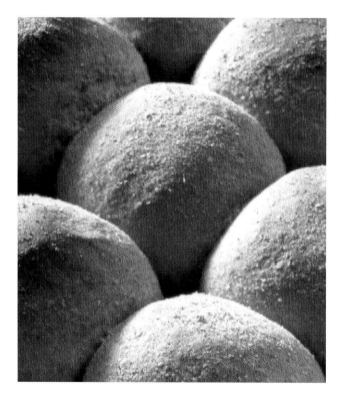

Eating wholemeal bread is much healthier than processed white bread.

THE VALUE OF FIBRE

Our bodies cannot digest some of the food that we eat, and it is this indigestible material that is known as dietary fibre – it comprises the walls of plant cells. But even though fibre cannot be considered a nutrient, it has a considerable impact on your health. For example, it has now been shown (after some previous inconclusive studies) that increasing your fibre intake to the recommended level of between 20 and 35 grams a day (most people eat considerably less than this), as part of an overall healthy diet, can significantly reduce the risk of developing cancer of the bowel (see page 13).

That is not all. Such a diet also reduces the acid levels in your stomach, which cause heartburn and gastro-oesophogal reflux disease, by up to 20 per cent. And importantly, it significantly reduces the risk of you developing heart disease and diabetes and suffering a stroke. This happens because one type of fibre can also lower the levels of cholesterol in your blood – which will lower your blood pressure (see page 8) and reduce your risk of developing other cancers, too.

There are two types of fibre: insoluble and soluble (the latter is so-called because it forms a gel when mixed with liquid). Insoluble fibre plays the main part in promoting bowel function and protecting against bowel cancer, and high levels of it are found in foods such as wholemeal bread, wheat cereals, rice, barley, grains, cabbage, carrots and so on. But it is soluble fibre that reduces blood cholesterol – though it is not clear how it does this. It is found in oats, oat bran, oatmeal, peas, beans, barley and fruits, and, conveniently, foods containing soluble fibre have a low GI rating (see page 17).

Five a day

So it makes sense to increase your intake of foods rich in fibre, and especially of those rich in soluble fibre – generally, it is recommended that you should eat five portions of fibre-rich fruit and vegetables a day. Make sure that you read labels carefully, though, because some commercial products that claim to be rich in fibre in fact contain very little of it.

Gently does it

Until your digestive system becomes accustomed to a high-fibre diet, you may find that it causes some disconcerting side-effects, such as wind and bloating. Constipation can be a problem, too, because fibre absorbs water.

The answer is to introduce your new diet gradually. Try swapping one group of low-fibre foods for high-fibre ones at a time – wholegrain bread for white processed bread, for example, then bran flakes for cornflakes. And make sure that you drink plenty of water.

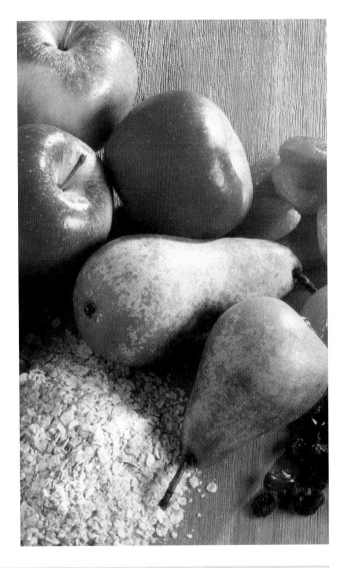

TAKE MEDICAL ADVICE

Always consult your doctor before adopting a new diet regime. Many diets are unsuitable for people who suffer from certain conditions or are taking medication. In particular, a high-fibre diet may not be suitable for people who have a condition called diverticulitis, in which the wall of the bowel becomes inflamed.

A HEALTHY DIET

A high-fibre diet does have many health advantages, but cannot, on its own, be said to constitute a healthy diet. In the following pages, we are going to explore the link between nutrition and disease and show how you can improve your health by changing your diet. Essentially, it limits your intake of certain carbohydrates and fats, and maximizes your intake of life-preserving, high-fibre vegetables, fruits and grains.

Diet and blood pressure

Most people know that high blood pressure puts the whole circulatory system at risk, causing a build-up of fatty plaques in the arteries and leading to heart disease or a stroke. What is less well known is that it is also a risk factor for certain cancers – in particular, for kidney cancer. But what is high blood pressure and what causes it?

Pressure points

The phrase 'high blood pressure' means that the force that blood exerts on the walls of arteries as it flows through them is higher than is normal. Blood pressure values are expressed as two figures, representing millimetres of mercury in an old-fashioned blood pressure measuring device (a sphygmomanometer): 120/80, for example, is considered normal – the first figure is the systolic pressure, when the heart is pumping; the second is the diastolic pressure, when the heart is resting between beats. You are considered to have high blood pressure, and will be offered treatment for it, if your reading is 140/90 or higher. It is estimated that between 10 and 20 per cent of the population have high blood pressure, but many people do not know that they have it – there are often no symptoms, which is why it is sometimes known as 'the silent killer'.

Atherosclerosis is the condition in which plaques (atheromata) form on the inner walls of arteries. The plaques consist of dead cells, fibrous tissue and calcium, among other things, but primarily contain cholesterol. They can cause the arteries to harden, narrow and become less flexible (arteriosclerosis), or block them. If atherosclerosis blocks the coronary arteries, which supply the heart with blood, the result will be a heart attack. Sometimes, too, pieces of plaque can break off (thrombi) and be carried around the circulatory system to block other, smaller blood vessels – if these supply blood to the brain, the result could be a stroke.

FOODS TO CHOOSE
(High in soluble fibre)
Oatmeal and *oat bran*
Lentils, beans and *peas*
Apples, bananas, blueberries, oranges, pears and *strawberries*
Sweetcorn, spinach, spring greens and *broccoli*
Nuts – almonds, brazil, cashews, hazel, peanuts, pecan, pistachio and walnuts
Seeds – sesame, sunflower and pumpkin

KEEP CHECKING

There are often no symptoms if you have high blood pressure – which is why it is known as the silent killer. But it is important that you know what your blood pressure is, so that you can take steps to reduce it if it is too high. In Britain, it is recommended that everybody asks their family doctor to check their blood pressure every five years, and more frequently with age; in the US, the recommendation is that blood pressure should be checked every two years over the age of 20.

The nature of the link between atherosclerosis and high blood pressure is complex. Each condition can cause the other one, but generally both develop as a result of lifestyle factors and the natural processes of aging (some people also have an inherited predisposition to them). Smoking, drinking excessive amounts of alcohol, obesity, high stress levels and the presence of other conditions, such as diabetes, play a major part in the development of both problems, but so, too, does your diet.

The culprits

The main dietary culprits when it comes to developing atherosclerosis and high blood pressure – and so some cancers – are saturated fats, trans fats, dietary cholesterol and salt. But some foods can actually prevent both problems. The trick is to know which foods to choose and which to avoid – and what follows will show you.

FOODS TO USE

(High in insoluble fibre)

Whole grains – bran, wheat, couscous, brown rice, bulgur and barley

wholemeal and *granary bread*

wholemeal pasta

wholemeal flour

Wholegrain breakfast cereals

Fruit – both fresh and dried

All vegetables – but especially Brussels sprouts, carrots, cabbage, okra, parsnips, sweetcorn, courgettes, cucumber, celery, tomatoes and unpeeled potatoes

FIBRE SUPPLEMENTS

Avoid commercially available fibre supplements, such as guar gum and cellulose. Not only are these expensive, but concerns have been expressed about their possible side-effects; also they do not seem to be effective at helping weight loss. It is far better to take your fibre the natural way.

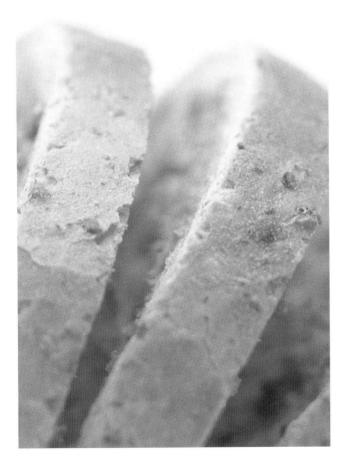

HIGH FIBRE EQUALS WEIGHT LOSS

There are a number of reasons why you lose weight on a high fibre diet. High-fibre foods:

- require more chewing, so you eat more slowly
- have extra bulk, so you feel full more quickly
- empty more slowly from the stomach, so you feel full for longer
- have fewer calories, so you feel full but have fewer to burn off.

FATS AND CHOLESTEROL

For many years, scientists believed that the cholesterol that you eat is the villain of the piece when it comes to heart disease. In fact, about 75 per cent of the cholesterol in your blood is manufactured by your liver, while only 25 per cent of it is in your diet. And the liver uses dietary fat to make cholesterol. When this was appreciated, the emphasis moved to eating a low-fat and low-cholesterol diet. But then it was discovered that it is not only the amount of fat in your diet that is important, but how much of which type of fat you eat – and there are three main types of fat: saturated fats, unsaturated fats and trans fats.

Saturated fats are found in meat, poultry, lard and whole-milk dairy products, such as cheese, milk, butter and cream, but high levels are also found in some vegetable oils, such as coconut and palm oil.

Unsaturated fats, which typically are liquid at room temperature, are found in plant and vegetable oils, such as olive, peanut, sesame, safflower, corn, sunflower, canola and soybean oil, and in avocados, oily fish (in the form or omega –3 fatty acid) and nuts and seeds.

Trans fats are man-made – a by-product of heating vegetable oils in the presence of hydrogen (which is why they are often referred to as 'hydrogenated vegetable oils' on product labels). They are found in commercially baked goods, such as biscuits; snack foods; processed foods; and commercially prepared fried foods, such as crisps. Some margarines also contain high levels of trans fats, especially brands that are 'stick' margarines – spreadable ones have less high levels as they are less hydrogenated (hydrogenation makes the fat hard at room temperature).

Where cholesterol comes in

Your body needs cholesterol to function correctly – it is involved in the production of hormones, the body's chemical messengers, as well as bile and vitamin D, and is found in every part of the body. For this reason, it is manufactured in the liver – and the liver uses fats to make it. If you eat too much saturated fat, the liver produces too much cholesterol. And, unfortunately, cholesterol is a soft, waxy substance that can stick to the lining of blood vessels and obstruct them if there are high levels of it in the blood.

As we have seen, liver-produced cholesterol, and so the cholesterol that is ultimately the result of fat consumption, accounts for around 75 per cent of the cholesterol found in you blood. The remaining 25 per cent comes from the cholesterol you eat. Dietary cholesterol is found in eggs, dairy products, meat, poultry, fish and shellfish, but the highest levels are found in egg yolks, meats such as liver and kidneys and shellfish. Vegetables, fruits, nuts, grains and cereals contain no cholesterol.

'Good' and 'bad' cholesterol

Cholesterol is carried around the body by chemicals called lipoproteins. There are two types: low-density lipoprotein (LDL) and high-density lipoprotein (HDL). If there is too much of the cholesterol carried by LDL, known as 'bad' cholesterol, plaque builds up on arterial walls. But HDL carries cholesterol away from the arteries to the liver, which breaks it down so that it can be excreted from the body; for this reason, HDL cholesterol is said to be 'good' cholesterol. It is now known that saturated fats, and, in particular, trans fats, increase the blood levels of harmful LDL cholesterol and lower levels of beneficial HDL cholesterol, while unsaturated fats have the opposite effect.

To sum up, then, a healthy diet, which helps prevent heart disease and some cancers, is one that has low levels of saturated and trans fats, and high levels of unsaturated fats – and, of course, is high in fibre.

FOODS TO USE SPARINGLY

(Rich in dietary cholesterol)

Organ meats – liver and kidneys

Eggs (especially ones from battery-farmed chickens)

Shellfish

Red meat

FOODS TO CHOOSE

(Containing unsaturated fat)

Vegetable oils – pure olive, peanut, walnut, sesame, corn, soybean, sunflower and safflower oils

Avocados

Oily fish – salmon, mackerel, tuna, herrings and so on

Nuts and seeds

Spreadable, unsaturated margarine

FOODS TO USE SPARINGLY

(Containing saturated fat)

Whole-fat milk (skimmed milk is preferable)

Butter, cream, cheese, full-fat yoghurt (low-fat is preferable), ice cream

Meat – beef, lamb and pork

Poultry – battery-farmed chicken (free-range is preferable), goose, duck and turkey (wild game, such as rabbit, wild duck and venison, is better)

Lard

Eggs (especially ones from battery-farmed chickens)

Coconut oil and palm oil

FOODS TO AVOID

(Containing trans fats)

Ready-made commercial foods – cakes, biscuits and snack foods

Processed foods – sausages, pâté, scotch eggs, pies and so on

Commercially prepared fried foods – crisps, pre-packaged, battered fish and chips

Hard margarine

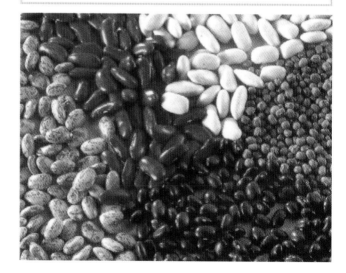

SALT

The more salt you eat, the more your body retains fluid, and the more fluid there is, the harder your heart has to work to pump blood around your body. And the result of this increase in the heart's work rate is high blood pressure and the risk, over time, of developing heart failure. High levels of salt in your diet are also linked to the incidence of certain cancers – in particular to stomach cancer.

Doctors recommend that our daily intake of salt should be less than 6 grams – about a teaspoonful. Even less salt than this is recommended for those who already have heart problems. The level is lower for children, too: up to 6 months old, it is less than 1 gram; between 7 and 12 months it is 1 gram; between 1 and 3 years it is 2 grams; between 4 and 6 it is 3 grams; and between 7 and 10 years it is 5 grams. Worryingly, one small can of spaghetti hoops served on a piece of toast made from white, supermarket bread contains around 0.9 grams – half of a toddler's recommended daily intake.

Hidden salt

The 6 gram target sounds an easy enough one to achieve, but in fact it is a very tall order. The reason is that this target refers to our total salt intake, not just to the salt that we add to our food, and there is a considerable amount of salt hidden in the foods many of us eat. Processed foods are mainly to blame – in fact, researchers estimate that around 75 per cent of our salt intake comes from them.

It is obvious that some foods contain high salt levels: salted nuts, crisps, olives and anchovies, for example, all taste, and are, salty. But bacon, cheese, pickles, stock cubes, sausages and smoked meat and fish contain salt, too. And some brands of biscuits, pizzas, 'ready meals', soups and breakfast cereals are also surprisingly high in salt.

The only way to check which processed foods are high in salt is to read product labels carefully. It is easy to come unstuck when you do this, however, because some labels do not refer to the product's salt content but to its sodium content (salt is made up of sodium and chloride). The two values are not the same – in fact, you have to multiply the sodium value by 2.5 to obtain the real salt content.

Reducing your salt intake

If you cut down on salt, your blood pressure will fall within weeks, even if it was not too high in the first place. And that means that your risk of developing heart disease, having a stroke or developing certain cancers will also fall.

Many people think that their food will lack taste if they cut down on salt, but this is a myth. You may find that your diet is a little bland for the first week or so, but your taste buds soon adapt. Adopt these salt reduction strategies and you will find the process much more easy.

- **Avoid** processed foods
- **Check** the salt levels of all commercially prepared foods, including everyday products such as bread
- **Throw** away your salt shaker
- **Make** your own salt-free stocks and sauces
- **Use** alternative seasonings, such as lemon juice, herbs and vinegar
- **Eat** fresh fruit (bananas and avocados in particular) and vegetables: the potassium they contain helps counter the effect of dietary salt
- **Do not** switch to sea salt, rock salt or garlic salt – they are not different to normal salt
- **Ask** your doctor whether salt substitutes are suitable for you.

FOODS TO AVOID

All types of salt – table, rock, sea and garlic
Obviously salty foods – anchovies, salted nuts and ready-salted crisps

FOODS TO USE SPARINGLY

(High in salt)
Commercially made foods – biscuits, supermarket bread, cheese biscuits and crisps
Ready-made meals – including pasta, pizzas, curries and Asian cuisine
Tinned foods – baked beans, spaghetti, meats and vegetables

Preserved and smoked foods – bacon, ham, pickles, spiced sausage, stock cubes and sauces

---

CALCULATE YOUR SALT INTAKE

If you must eat processed foods – and it can be hard not to – try to make sure that you stay within the recommended daily intake of 6 grams of salt. Read a product's label to find the number of grams of salt in 100 grams of the contents. If the quantity of sodium is given, multiply by 2.5 to calculate the actual salt content. (If the value is given in milligrams, or 'mg', divide by 1,000 to convert it to grams.)

Then look for the total weight of the contents, or estimate the proportion of them that you intend to use. Divide the weight that you will use by 100, then multiply by the number of grams of salt in each 100 grams and you will discover how much salt you will eat.

Grapefruit can be used to make a great salt substitute

SALT SUBSTITUTES

Some people find that their food tastes a little bland when they switch to a low-salt diet, and even though their taste buds will adapt within a few weeks some people find that they need a little help to make the change. A number of salt substitutes are on the market, but these contain part sodium and part potassium and in certain circumstances it is possible to overload your body with potassium – consult your doctor before using a commercial salt substitute.

Make your own

This recipe for a salt substitute relies on the principle that a sour flavour is a good substitute for a salty one. It uses the grapefruit peel (or lemon or orange peel, for a weaker taste) and citric acid crystals. Also known as 'sour salt' and "lemon salt", these can be found in the baking section of supermarkets or in delicatessens.

Ingredients

The peel of 1 grapefruit
1 tbsp ground allspice
$1/2$ tbsp citric acid crystals

Makes 3 tablespoons

Method

1 Peel the grapefruit as thinly as possible, then scrape away all the white parts. Dry the peel overnight near a source of heat.

2 Grind the dried peel in a coffee grinder or spice grinder, then combine it with the other ingredients. Put the mixture into a well-sealed bottle and shake well to mix. Store in a dry place.

Variations

Add a tablespoon of freshly ground black pepper to the mixture to make it into citrus pepper, an ideal seasoning for meat.

DIET AND CANCER

Contrary to popular belief, carcinogens (cancer-causing chemicals) in the diet are only very rarely a cause of cancer. The 15-year analysis of statistics relating to food intake and diet undertaken by the AICR has demonstrated that in a hugely significant proportion of cancer cases, the changes are the result of eating an unhealthy diet. Unfortunately, nobody knows for certain why this should be – perhaps ongoing research will provide the answer.

Here is a summary of the main findings of the AICR's study linking a reduction in the risks of specific cancers to dietary measures – as you will see, high-fibre vegetables and fruit are preventive against a number of types of cancer:

- **Lung cancer**: the most common cause of lung cancer is tobacco smoking, but a diet rich in vegetables and fruits may prevent between 20 and 33 per cent of cases in both smokers and non-smokers

- **Stomach cancer**: diets high in vegetables and fruits, and low in salt, together with the routine use of freezing and refrigeration of perishable foods may prevent between 66 and 75 per cent of cases

- **Breast cancer**: a diet rich in vegetables and fruit, an appropriate body weight and an avoidance of alcohol may prevent between 10 and 20 per cent of cases (more if this diet is adopted early in life)

- **Bowel cancer**: a diet high in fibre and vegetables and low in meat and alcohol may, together with regular physical exercise, prevent between 66 and 75 per cent of cases

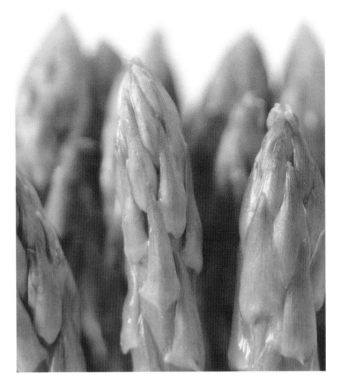

Eating a healthy amount of fruit and vegetables has been linked to a reduced risk of developing some cancers.

- **Mouth and throat cancer**: a diet high in vegetables and fruit, and low in alcohol consumption may – in the absence of tobacco smoking – prevent between 30 and 50 per cent of cases

- **Liver cancer**: avoidance of alcohol (and of aflatoxins, found in a mould that grows on some nuts) may prevent between 33 and 66 per cent of cases.

The message seems fairly clear: if you smoke, stop now; moderate your alcohol intake; cut down on the amount of meat you eat; and emphasize high-fibre vegetables and fruits in your diet. And it is particularly important that you take these steps if you have a family history of cancer, because genetic predisposition is a major risk factor for developing cancer.

Luckily, an anti-cancer diet is the same as the diet that doctors and nutritionists recommend for healthy living – and it is a high-fibre diet, too – and it is this same diet that can prevent numerous other conditions, such as high blood pressure, heart disease and diabetes. It relies on limiting your intake of certain carbohydrates and fats, and maximizing your intake of life-preserving, high-fibre vegetables, fruits and grains. In the following pages we will show you how to do just that – starting with a look at the chemicals, obtainable in a healthy diet, that actually prevent cancer from developing.

ANTIOXIDANTS, VITAMINS AND MINERALS

Many of our bodily structures can be damaged by the presence of what are known as 'free radicals' – technically speaking, these are atoms that have unpaired electrons. The most common free radical is radical oxygen, which can damage cells, causing them to develop cancerous changes, and increase the likelihood that cholesterol forms fatty plaques in arteries, leading to heat disease.

When this was realized, in the 1990s, nutritionists started to look at the antioxidants that combat radical oxygen and so help prevent cancer and heart disease. These are known as 'phytochemicals', which literally means 'plant chemicals', and the most important antioxidants amongst them are vitamins C and E, beta-carotene (a precursor to vitamin A) and lycopene. Soon antioxidant supplements became increasingly popular, and today some 30 per cent of Americans take them. Unfortunately, they do not reduce the risks of cancer, heart disease or stroke, as a series of studies, and meta-studies (that is, studies of studies) have shown.

Nevertheless, it has been shown that a diet that is high in antioxidants is protective against cancer and heart disease. The answer to this conundrum is thought to be that in practice the effect of dietary antioxidants relies on the interaction between the antioxidants and other dietary ingredients: minerals, perhaps, or fibre. So it is important to eat a diet rich in antioxidants – that means richly coloured fruit and vegetables that contain chemicals called flavonoids, such as apricots, blueberries, bilberries, broccoli, carrots, mangos, peppers and spinach, and, in particular, tomatoes (though these should be cooked to release maximum quantities of flavonoids). And, just to show that a healthy diet need not be without its luxuries, there are high levels of flavonoids in both dark chocolate and red wine – though both should be enjoyed in moderation.

VITAMINS AND MINERALS

Every one of our body's systems need vitamins and minerals to function. Vitamins act as catalysts, initiating and controlling chemical reactions in the body, while minerals also play a vital part in body chemistry. Only small amounts of them are needed – they are known as micronutrients – and they must be obtained from our diet, because the body cannot manufacture them. If you follow the rules for healthy eating given in this book, and take a multivitamin supplement every day, as a precaution, you should absorb all the vitamins and minerals that your body requires. (Doing so is particularly important on a high-fibre diet, since it can reduce the amount of some vitamins and minerals – calcium in particular – absorbed in the intestines.) But sometimes the way that we treat and cook food reduces its content of micronutrients. Follow these rules to make sure that you can meet your body's requirements.

- Avoid processed foods, and canned foods in particular, because these can be low in vitamin content.

- Always use fresh or frozen fruit and vegetables, because vitamin levels decrease as these foods age. It is not generally realized that freezing preserves vitamin content, but chilling fruit and vegetables in a refrigerator before heating them can reduce levels of vitamins such as vitamin C and folic acid by up to 30 per cent. Remember that frozen vegetables – peas, especially – are often more vitamin-rich than fresh ones, because they are frozen immediately after being picked.

- **Keep** all foods away from heat, light and air, all of which reduce levels of vitamin C and the B vitamins. Store vegetables in airtight bags.

- **Use** the skin of fruits and vegetables wherever possible and avoid trimming them too much. Instead of peeling, wash or scrub them – most of the nutritional value of fruits and vegetables is contained in the skin or the area underneath it.

- **Keep** the water you have used to cook vegetables and use it as a base for stocks or sauces – otherwise you will lose the valuable vitamins and minerals that have leached into the water.

- **Take** a daily multivitamin supplement – it can be hard to obtain sufficient quantities of some vitamins, such as B12 and folic acid from your diet; and fibre-rich foods contain chemicals called phytates, which can bind with some minerals and interfere with their absorption. But think of it as a nutritional safety net, rather than as a substitute for healthy eating.

VITAMIN– AND MINERAL–RICH FOODS

(NB Pre-menopausal women and women taking HRT should eat more of foods containing vitamins that are depleted by the female hormone oestrogen.)

Vitamin A (antioxidant)
Retinol: butter, cod liver oil and cheese
Beta-carotene: apricots, cantaloupe, carrots, kale, peach, peas, spinach and sweet potatoes

Vitamin B1
Beans, brown rice, milk, oatmeal, vegetables, whole grains and yeast (depleted by alcohol, caffeine, exposure to air and water, food additives and oestrogen)

Vitamin B2
Eggs, fish, meat, milk, vegetables and whole grains (depleted by alcohol, caffeine, oestrogen and zinc)

Vitamin B3
Avocado, eggs, fish, meat, peanuts, prunes, seeds and whole grains (destroyed by canning and some sleeping pills; depleted by alcohol and oestrogen)

Vitamin B5
Bran, eggs, green vegetables, meat, whole grains and yeast (destroyed by canning)

Vitamin B6
Avocado, bananas, cabbage, cantaloupe, fish, milk, eggs, seeds and wheat bran (destroyed by alcohol, heat, oestrogen and processing techniques during production of commercial food)

Vitamin B folic acid
Apricots, avocados, beans, carrots, green vegetables, melons, oranges and whole wheat (destroyed by commercial food processing techniques, cooking and exposure to water and air, depleted by alcohol)

Vitamin B12
Dairy products, fish and meat (depleted by alcohol, exposure to sunlight and water, oestrogen and sleeping tablets)

Vitamin C (antioxidant)
Broccoli, cabbage, cauliflower, citrus fruits, green peppers, spinach, tomatoes and potatoes (destroyed by boiling, exposure to air, and carbon dioxide and long storage; depleted by alcohol, aspirin, oestrogen, stress and tobacco)

Vitamin D
Cod liver oil, dairy products and oily fish (depleted by lack of sunlight)

Vitamin E (antioxidant)
Almonds, broccoli, eggs, kale, oats, olive oil, peanuts, soybeans, seeds, spinach and wheat germ (destroyed by commercial food processing techniques, freezing, heat, oxygen and chlorine; depleted by smoking and use of contraceptive pills)

Vitamin K
Broccoli, cod liver oil, eggs, green vegetables, live yoghurt, tomatoes and whole grains

Magnesium
Bitter chocolate, brown rice, nuts, soybeans and wholewheat (depleted by caffeine and stress)

Zinc (antioxidant)
Eggs, meat, mushrooms, yeast and whole grains (inhibited by caffeine and smoking)

Potassium
Avocados, bananas, dried fruit, green vegetables, nuts and potatoes (lost in diarrhoea and sweat)

Selenium (antioxidant)
Broccoli, onions, tomatoes, tuna and wheat germ

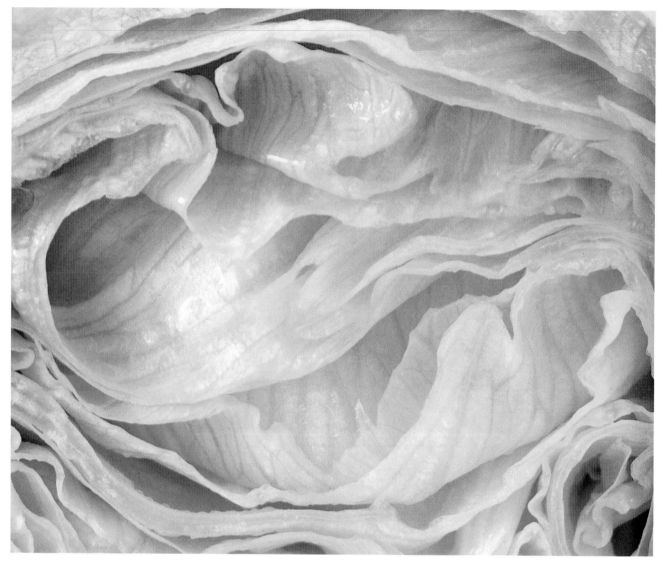

Lettuce is a great side to any meal,
and is a good source of vitamin A and C.

TOO MUCH CAN BE DANGEROUS

Many people take high doses of vitamin supplements, without having taken medical advice. But doing so can be dangerous, because in many cases the effects of high doses are not known, and in some cases the effects have been confirmed to be dangerous. For example, it was once thought that very high doses of vitamin E might help prevent heart disease, but several studies have failed to show this and a recent study suggests that they may make heart failure more likely. And the list goes on: too much calcium can lead to lethargy, confusion and coma; excess vitamin B6 can cause a nerve disorder that leads to loss of feeling in the arms and legs; too much beta-carotene can increase the risk of contracting lung cancer in smokers; high doses of vitamin A can increase the risk of cardiovascular disease and can damage your liver; excessive doses of vitamin C can cause abdominal pain, nausea and diarrhoea; and so on.

The message is clear: do not take high-dose vitamin supplements unless they have been prescribed by your doctor – you can obtain all the antioxidants, vitamins and minerals you need by eating a healthy diet and taking a daily multivitamin and mineral supplement.

CARBOHYDRATES

Carbohydrates are the body's primary source of fuel and are an essential part of a healthy diet. There are three types of carbohydrate: sugars, fibre and starch, and all of them are built from molecules of sugar. They used to be described as 'complex' or 'simple' carbohydrates, depending on whether they were simple forms of sugar or consisted of linked forms of sugar, and it was believed that simple carbohydrates should be avoided and complex ones preferred.

Today this categorization is now longer used. Instead, nutritionists classify carbohydrates according to their glycaemic index, or 'GI'. During the digestive process, carbohydrates are broken down into the simplest forms of sugar, and the glycaemic index measures how quickly this happens and so how fast levels of sugar in the blood rise – a high GI value means that the carbohydrate raises these levels very quickly.

The significance of this is that the pancreas starts to produce the hormone insulin in response to rising blood sugar levels, and this promotes the uptake of sugar by the body's cells and reduces sugar levels in the blood. If you continually eat foods with a high GI – and if you have a hereditary disposition to the problem or are overweight and inactive – the levels of both insulin and sugar in your blood remain high, and you develop what is known as insulin resistance (the body loses its sensitivity to insulin, so more and more is needed). This can not only lead to type 2 diabetes, but result in high blood pressure, low levels of 'good' cholesterol (see page 10) and the risk of heart disease.

There is some evidence that eating high GI carbohydrates may also be linked to an increased risk of colorectal, breast and pancreatic cancer, though the link has not been conclusively proved as yet. Until more is known, though, it would be sensible to choose a diet that emphasizes low and medium GI foods.

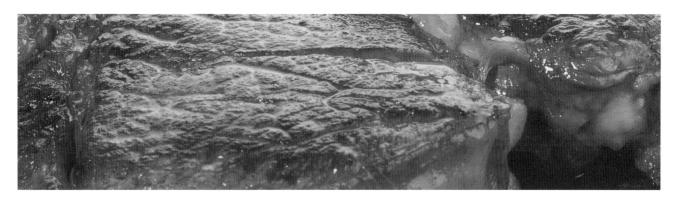

HIGH OR LOW?

In essence, whether a food has a high or low GI depends on how quickly its carbohydrates are converted to simple sugar during the digestive process. Foods that have not been processed – whole-grain foods – still contain their original fibre, which slows down the rate at which carbohydrates are converted to simple sugars and so also slows down the rate at which sugar enters the bloodstream; conversely, the carbohydrates in processed foods have already been partly broken down, meaning that their sugar enters the bloodstream relatively quickly.

However, the type of starch in the food is important, too: potatoes, for example, contain a starch that is broken down quickly during digestion. Other factors affecting the GI value are: ripeness – ripe fruit has a higher GI than unripe fruit; acidity – vinegar and lemon juice delay stomach emptying and so reduce the

GI value; and the size of food particles – small particles are more easily absorbed and increase the GI value.

High-fibre foods have a low GI value, but low GI foods also include foods such as soy and milk; medium ones include sugar, orange juice and oats; while high GI foods include potatoes, rice, and wholemeal and white bread. It might seem a daunting prospect to exist solely on low GI foods, but it is not necessary to do so. This is because eating a low GI food reduces the GI value of high GI foods when they are eaten at the same time – if, for example, you eat cornflakes (high GI) with milk (low GI) your blood sugar levels will not go up as quickly – what is known as the overall "glycaemic load" (GL) is reduced. In essence, the equation reads "high GI + low GI = medium GI." So if you plan your menus carefully you can still eat some high GI foods.

PLUSES AND A MINUS

Maximizing the amount of low GI foods in your diet and minimizing the amount of high GI ones has numerous benefits:

- the slow breakdown of low GI foods during digestion and the gradual release of their sugars into your bloodstream means that you will not feel the 'sugar let-down' that comes when quick-release sugars are used up; in turn this means that you will not need to have another 'sugar hit' as quickly, so you will eat less – which means that you will lose weight (about ½ to 1 kg a week)

- the slow release of sugars into your bloodstream increases your physical endurance

- a low GI diet increases the body's sensitivity to insulin, which reduces the risk of developing insulin resistance, and so diabetes and heart disease

- including a larger proportion of low GI foods means that you will reduce your intake of 'bad' saturated fats and trans fats (see page 9) and lessen the likelihood that you will develop heart disease

- there is some evidence that a low GI diet may help prevent some cancers

- so long as you choose low GI foods, you can snack between meals

- a low GI diet leads to increased levels of serotonin in the brain – and serotonin makes you feel good

- a low GI diet can easily be followed for life, unlike other fad diets.

But, in case low-GI diet seems too good to be true, there is just one minus:

- healthy though they may be, even low GI foods contain calories, so if you eat too many of them you will not lose weight: you still have to control portion sizes.

FOODS TO CHOOSE
(Low glycaemic index carbohydrates)
Bran and *porridge oats*
Barley, buckwheat and *bulgur wheat*
Some fruits – apples, citrus, berries, peaches, pears, plums and rhubarb
Pasta
Some vegetables – avocados, aubergines, beans (runner and green), broccoli, cabbage, cauliflower, carrots, celery, courgettes, cucumber, leeks, onions, lettuce, mushrooms, olives, peas, peppers, spinach and tomatoes

FOODS TO USE SPARINGLY
(Medium glycaemic index carbohydrates)
Pure wheat cereals
Granary and *wholemeal bread*
Basmati or *long-grained rice, wild rice* and *couscous*
Corn – cornmeal, corn oil and sweetcorn
Some fruits – apricots, bananas, melon, dried fruit, pineapples mangos
Some vegetables – new potatoes, sweet potatoes, beetroot and artichokes
Honey

FOODS TO AVOID
(High glycaemic index carbohydrates)
Breakfast cereals – *cornflakes and sugar-coated cereals*
White bread, cakes, biscuits, bagels, buns, muffins, pancakes and *doughnuts*
White and *brown rice*
Some fruits – dates, prunes and watermelon
Gnocchi
Some vegetables – broad beans, potatoes (when mashed, baked, fried or roasted), parsnips and swede
Sugar – table, glucose, treacle and molasses
Tomato ketchup

PROTEIN

Protein, made up from chemicals called amino acids, make up the building blocks of all our body's tissues except stored fat. You need to eat a certain amount of protein every day – a minimum of one gram for every kilogram of body weight – to prevent the body from starting to break down tissue. And you need more than that if you want to build up healthy muscles and bones. It is easy to get enough protein in your diet in Western industrialized societies, though hard to do so in developing countries. But the quantity of protein you eat is not the whole story. What is important is that you eat a variety of amino acids, which means protein from a variety of sources. This does not mean that it is essential to eat steaks, for example, because you can obtain a full range of proteins from vegetable and fruit sources, if you are a vegetarian. Variety is the watchword.

THE DANGERS OF BEING OVERWEIGHT

Being overweight brings with it the dangers of many health problems, including an increased risk of developing colonic and rectal cancer, but if you carry the extra pounds on your waist – in the classic 'beer belly' – you are far more at risk of heart disease or diabetes. In fact, men with waists of more than 101cm (40 inches) and women with waists of more than 89cm (35 inches) are at between double and quadruple the risk of developing them.

The reason is that fat that is stored around the stomach secretes hormones that play havoc with the production of insulin, the pancreatic hormone that controls blood sugar levels. As a result 'insulin resistance' develops, leading to diabetes, high blood pressure and high cholesterol levels. And a very successful – and healthy – way to lose weight is to adopt a high-fibre, low-fat diet.

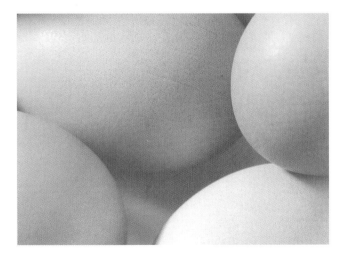

FOODS TO CHOOSE

('Good' protein – lower in saturated fats)

Vegetables – beans, brown rice, lentils, millet and pulses

Soybeans

Nuts – brazil, peanuts and pine-buts

Seeds – sesame

Free-range chicken and *turkey (but remove the skin)*

Locally sourced lean cuts of non-intensively reared meats – beef, lamb, pork and veal

Free-range chicken eggs (but not duck or goose eggs)

CHECK THE LABEL

Food manufacturers are starting to note GI values on product labels, and the practice is likely to become more and more widespread. (In fact, the World Health Authority advises that GI values should be stated and that the values for 'complex carbohydrates' and sugars, which are used currently, are dropped.) But how do you interpret the figures?

The answer is that the maximum GI value, which is based on pure glucose, is 100, and that foods are said to have a low GI when the value is 55 or less; to be medium GI when the value is between 56 and 69; and high GI when the value is 70 or more. Remember that, ideally, you should stick to low GI foods; failing that, your diet should combine medium and low GI foods; and that if you ever eat high GI foods you should combine them with low GI ones.

STRIKING A BALANCE

It is easy to decide which foods you should eat, but more difficult to decide how often to eat them. It is also hard to strike a nutritional balance between foods so that you obtain all the nutrients that your body demands in the correct quantities, yet protect your heart and arteries at the same time. And you will have noticed already from the tables in this book that certain foods are 'good' in the sense that they contain substantial quantities of a desirable ingredient, but 'not so good' in that they contain less desirable ingredients. So how do you do it?

The healthy eating pyramid shown on the opposite page indicates how often you should eat the different food groups. For instance, while certain foods are important as part of a balanced diet, they need to be eaten in moderation because of the health dangers associated with overindulgence.

As we have already seen, eating a balanced, nutritious diet that is high in fibre will yield many health benefits, and the recipes in this book demonstrate that high fibre food is also tasty and appetizing. Indeed, as will be demonstrated in the pages that follow, a high fibre diet is as delicious as it is healthy.

EXPLAINING THE SYMBOLS

SOLUBLE FIBRE

HIGH

MEDIUM

LOW

PROTEIN

HIGH

MEDIUM

LOW

ANTIOXIDANT

HIGH

MEDIUM

LOW

SATURATED FAT

HIGH

MEDIUM

LOW

UNSATURATED FAT

HIGH

MEDIUM

LOW

CHOLESTEROL

HIGH

MEDIUM

LOW

GLYCAEMIC INDEX

HIGH

MEDIUM

LOW

INSOLUBLE FIBRE

HIGH

MEDIUM

LOW

HEALTHY EATING PYRAMID

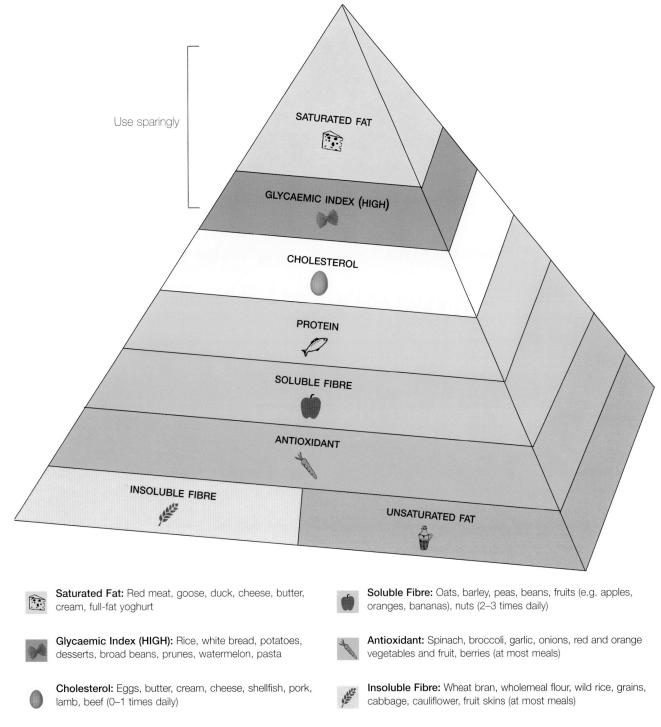

Saturated Fat: Red meat, goose, duck, cheese, butter, cream, full-fat yoghurt

Glycaemic Index (HIGH): Rice, white bread, potatoes, desserts, broad beans, prunes, watermelon, pasta

Cholesterol: Eggs, butter, cream, cheese, shellfish, pork, lamb, beef (0–1 times daily)

Protein: Fish, shellfish, free-range chicken, rabbit, wild game, low-fat dairy (1–2 times daily)

Soluble Fibre: Oats, barley, peas, beans, fruits (e.g. apples, oranges, bananas), nuts (2–3 times daily)

Antioxidant: Spinach, broccoli, garlic, onions, red and orange vegetables and fruit, berries (at most meals)

Insoluble Fibre: Wheat bran, wholemeal flour, wild rice, grains, cabbage, cauliflower, fruit skins (at most meals)

Unsaturated Fat: Olive oil, soya beans, avocado, peanuts, salmon, mackerel, tuna, sardines (1–2 times daily)

HOW TO COOK HEALTHILY

There is little point in choosing healthy ingredients and recipes if you cook them in a way that is in itself unhealthy. It is important to choose cooking methods that not only preserve fibre content, help reduce cholesterol and saturated fats and keep the calorie count low, but maximize the nutritional value of each dish. These techniques are effective, but may require a little practise:

- **Baking** – good for vegetables, fruit, poultry and lean meat, as well as for puddings; you may need a little extra liquid
- **Braising or stewing** – brown first, on top of the stove, then cook in a small quantity of liquid; if you leave the dish in a refrigerator you can remove the chilled fat and then reheat it
- **Grilling** – on a rack, so that fat can drain away, and not in a direct flame
- **Microwaving** – place the food between two paper towels to drain fat away while it cooks
- **Poaching** – in a covered pan of the correct size, so that you use the minimum liquid
- **Roasting** – on a rack so that the food does not sit in fat; baste with fat-free liquids, such as wine or lemon juice
- **Sautéing** – use a high heat and a small amount of non-stick cooking spray, or just cook without spray if you have a good-quality non-stick pan
- **Steaming** – in a perforated basket over simmering water; add seasoning to the water for extra flavour
- **Stir-frying** – in a wok, using a small amount of non-stick cooking spray or a tiny amount of olive oil.

You can also increase flavour, reduce fat and salt content and make the most of your ingredients' nutritional value if you

Remember to:

- Avoid cooking methods that char food, such as barbecuing or grilling over a direct flame – charring produces carcinogens
- Check labels for common ingredients, such as soy sauce, baking soda and monosodium glutamate – these all contain high levels of sodium and should be used very sparingly, if at all
- Make your own stock rather than using pre-prepared cubes, which can be high in salt
- Steam vegetables, for preference, in order to maximize both their flavour and nutritional value
- Cook lightly to preserve vitamin content (but cook meats and other foods that may harbour disease-producing organisms thoroughly)
- Choose extra virgin olive oil and vinegar rather than salted, pre-prepared salad dressings
- Wash canned vegetables before use – by doing so you can substantially reduce their salt content
- Use only one egg yolk when making scrambled eggs or omelettes, but mix in two or three extra egg whites
- Trim as much fat as you can from meat before you cook it and remove the skin from poultry
- Choose lean, low-fat meats, such as game (but, again, remember to remove the skin) and venison
- Drain oil from canned fish and rinse the fish in water before you use it
- Use herbs, wine, and freshly ground pepper to enhance flavours; remember that a dash of vinegar or lemon juice will not only enhance flavour but reduce the GI rating of other ingredients.

Steamed vegetables keep their full flavour and nuturitional value.

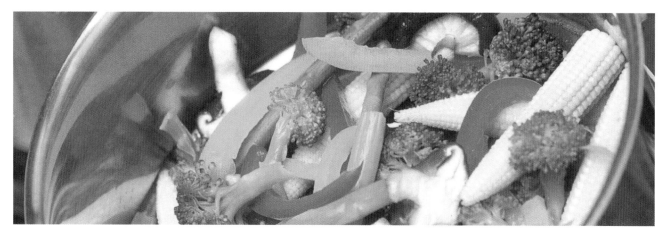

MAKE YOUR OWN STOCK

Many stock cubes contain high levels of salt and low levels of nutrients – and high salt levels are a risk factor for certain cancers, as well as increasing blood pressure. But nothing could be more simple than making your own stock, and if you make it in large batches you can freeze it for later use. You can use your stock as the basis for a delicious soup – serve it with a whole-grain roll – or as the basis of a nourishing stew or a piquant sauce.

FISH STOCK

Ingredients

1 kg fish bones, heads (with gills removed) and tails (sole or plaice are tastiest, but any other white, non-only fish will do)
1 large onion, coarsely chopped
2 shallots, coarsely chopped
2 ribs celery, tops included, coarsely chopped
2 large carrots, scrubbed but not peeled, coarsely chopped
2 bay leaves
2 cloves
6 sprigs parsley, coarsely chopped
1 Tbsp peppercorns
lemon rind from half a lemon
cold water to cover

Method

Place everything in a stockpot and bring to simmering point – do not allow to boil. Simmer for 20–30 minutes, but no longer or the stock will become bitter. Strain through cheesecloth or use a non-metallic colander. Reduce the strained stock by boiling, if required. Use or freeze as required.

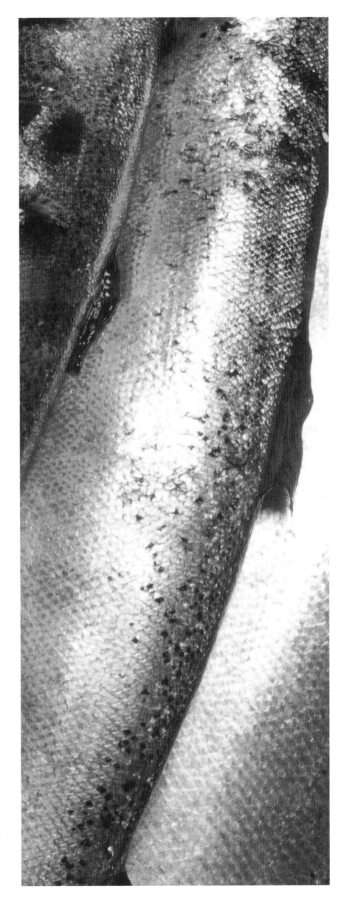

Oily fish is a great source of protein and natural oils, but can contain a large amount of calories.

VEGETABLE STOCK

Ingredients

3 large carrots, scrubbed but not peeled, coarsely
    chopped
1 turnip, coarsely chopped
2 onions, coarsely chopped
2 leeks, coarsely chopped
4 ribs celery, including tops, coarsely chopped
Coarsely chopped trimmings from cauliflour, spinach,
    broccoli or any other vegetables, so long as they are
    fresh and clean. Always use fresh vegetables.
1 cup any dried beans, having been soaked overnight,
    if necessary; or use rice or barley
2 tbsp olive oil
1 bouquet garni, which includes 3 sprigs parsley, 1
    sprig thyme and 1 bay leaf
1 tbsp peppercorns
Approx 3 litres cold water for 1 kg vegetables

Method

Warm the olive oil in a stockpot, add the vegetables
and simmer, stirring continuously for 15 minutes until
they start to colour slightly. Then add the water and
the other ingredients and bring to simmering point.
Simmer for at least 2 hours, adding more water if
necessary. Then strain through cheesecloth or use a
non-metallic colander. Use or freeze, as required.

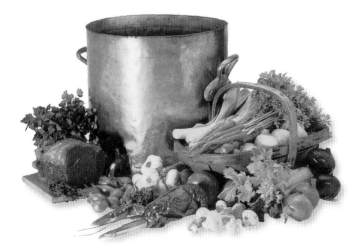

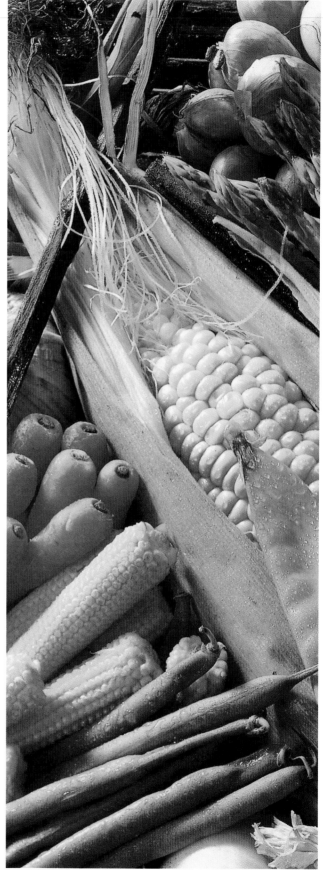

CHICKEN STOCK

Ingredients

The bones of a chicken, and, if available, a ham bone or a veal knuckle (ask your butcher for one)
2 leeks, coarsely chopped
2 large carrots, scrubbed but not peeled, coarsely chopped
3 large onions, coarsely chopped
2 ribs celery, tops included, coarsely chopped
6 sprigs parsley, coarsely chopped
1 large clove garlic
2 cloves
1 tbsp peppercorns
Lemon rind from half a lemon

Method

Place the bones in a stockpot and cover with cold water. Bring to simmering point – do not allow to boil. Simmer for at least an hour, then add all other ingredients and more cold water to cover, if necessary. Return to simmering point and simmer for another 2 hours. Then strain through cheesecloth or use a non-metallic colander. Refrigerate, and when stock has set remove any fat from the top. Use or freeze, as required.

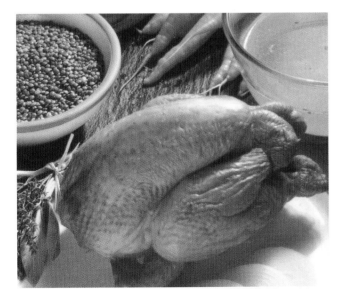

A HEALTHY LIFESTYLE

Eating a healthy diet is only one part of a healthy lifestyle. To reduce the risk of developing high blood pressure and some cancers, to lower cholesterol levels, promote cardiovascular health and improve the quality of your life, you should also:

Give up smoking

If you smoke, you are massively increasing the risk that you will develop lung, mouth or throat cancer, and more than doubling the risk of having a heart attack, as well as reducing the likelihood of surviving a heart attack

Manage stress

Use relaxation techniques and anger-management methods to cope with stress and keep your blood pressure low

Lose weight

If you are overweight, you are more at risk of developing certain cancers and between two and six times more likely to develop high blood pressure

Cut down on alcohol

There's evidence to suggest that two units of alcohol, and especially of red wine, can reduce blood pressure, but more than this can increase the risk of certain cancers and actually raise blood pressure

Lead an active life

Even small amounts of physical activity, for example walking or gardening, can increase the number of calories that you burn and so help lose weight, as well as reducing the risk of developing cancers and heart disease.

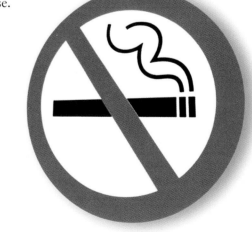

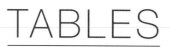

TABLES

These tables give the nutritional values for the main ingredients used in the recipes that follow. To eat healthily and minimize your risk of developing cancer, the major part of your diet should consist of foods with a high fibre content, a low fat content, moderate protein levels, a low or medium glycaemic index and with plenty of antioxidants. Use the Healthy Eating Pyramid on page 21 as a guide to proportions.

Remember that carrying excess weight is a major risk for developing ill health, so watch your calorie intake, too. Doctors recommend that men with a sedentary lifestyle – that of an office worker, say – should eat 2,700 calories a day, while women should eat 2,000. In order to lose weight gradually, at the rate of ½ kg a week, you need to reduce this figure by 500 calories.

Food	Quantity	Glycaemic index	Fat	Protein	Fibre	Calories
Meat and Dairy						
Cheese, feta	25 g	M	6	4	0	80
Cheese, reduced fat	25 g	M	4.5	7	0	70
Chicken skinless	100 g	L	5	30	0	150
Crème fraîche, low fat	100 g	M	17.5	3	0	800
Egg	1 medium	M	5.5	6	0	80
lean beef, lamb, pork	100 g	M	7	30	0	190
Milk, low fat	275 ml	L	2.5	8	0	102
Rabbit	100 g	L	4.5	30	0	160
Wild fowl	100 g	L	6	30	0	155
Yoghurt	100 g	L	0	5	0	40
Fish						
Herring, salmon	100 g	L	11	20	0	180
Mackerel	100 g	L	18	25	0	220
Sardine	100 g	L	2	15	0	65
Shellfish	100 g	L	1	15	0	105
Trout	100 g	L	6	20	0	155
Tuna	100 g	L	3	20	0	120
White fish	100 g	L	2	20	0	90

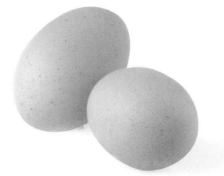

Dairy products such as eggs don't contain any fibre, and should be used sparingly.

Food	Quantity	Glycaemic index	Fat	Protein	Fibre	Calories
Fruit						
Apple	1 medium	L	0	0.5	2	45
Apricot	3	M	0	1.5	2	30
Banana	1 small	M	0.5	1	1	90
Berries, fresh	100 g	L	0	0.5	1	30
Dried fruit	50 g	M	0	0.5	4	80
Grapefruit	half	L	0	0.5	1	30
Melon	slice	M	0	0.5	1	50
Nectarine, peach	1 medium	L	0	0.5	1	35
Orange	1 medium	L	0	1.5	3	50

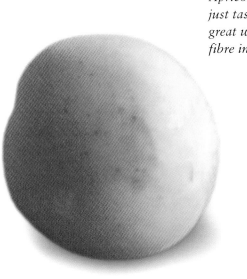

Apricots and apples don't just taste great but are great way to increase your fibre intake.

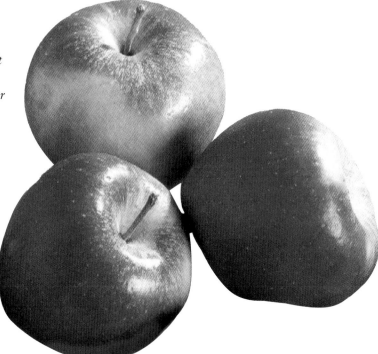

Food	Quantity	Glycaemic index	Fat	Protein	Fibre	Calories
Vegetables						
Avocado	½ medium	L	15	2	3.5	150
Beans	100 g	L	0.5	6	4	100
Beetroot	small	L	0	0.5	0.5	25
Broccoli	100 g	L	0	1.5	2.5	25
Cabbage	50 g	L	0	1	1	7
Carrot	50 g	L	0	0.5	1	12

Food	Quantity	Glycaemic index	Fat	Protein	Fibre	Calories
Vegetables *(continued)*						
Cauliflower	100 g	L	0	1	1.5	20
Aubergine	100 g	L	0	0.5	2	75
Green beans	100 g	L	0	1.5	2.5	20
Lettuce	medium	L	0	0.5	0.3	5
Onions	medium	L	0	1	1.4	30
Peas	100 g	L	0	3.5	6	60
Peppers	100 g	L	0	1	2.5	30
Potatoes, new	3	M	0	1.5	3	100
Soyabean	100 g	L	7	8	6	120
Spinach	60 g cooked	L	0	1	1	10
Squash, butternut	100 g	M	0	1	1.5	30
Sweetcorn	100 g	M	0.5	2.5	1.5	95
Tofu	100 g	L	4	8	0	70
Tomato	medium	L	0	1	1	15

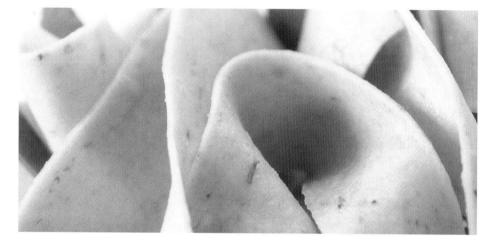

Foods such as pasta are seen as fattening, but it is the sauces, fats and oils added to the dish that are the culprits.

Food	Quantity	Glycaemic index	Fat	Protein	Fibre	Calories
Cereal, Nuts, Pulses						
Barley	50 g raw	L	1	2	1	140
Buckwheat	100 g	L	2.5	3	2.1	330
Chickpeas	100 g	L	3	5	4	110
Cornstarch	100 g	M	0.7	2	0.1	350
Lentils	100 g	L	0.5	8	2	100
Oats	50 g raw	L	1	4	3	140
Pasta, wholegrain	100 g	L	1	5	4	120
Rice, brown, basmati	100 g	M	0	3.5	1	200
Walnuts	2 Tbsp	L	8	2	1	80
Wild rice	100 g	M	0	3	1	100

BREAKFASTS

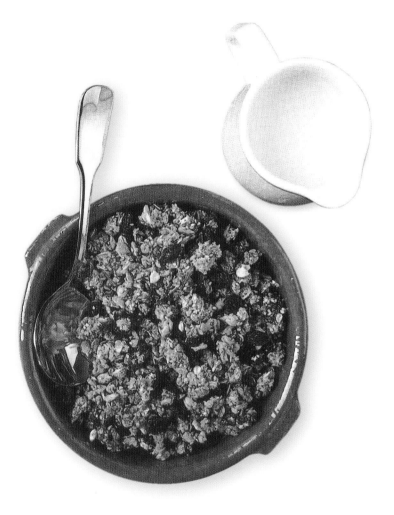

PRUNE VELVET

SERVES **4**

A very fruity start to the day is to be had with this high fibre breakfast dish.

225 g pitted no-need-to-soak prunes

8 tbsp orange juice

1 tsp clear honey

1 tbsp dark brown muscovado sugar

300 ml low-fat natural yoghurt

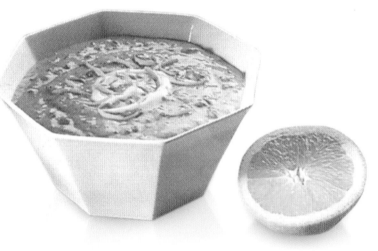

1 Place the prunes and orange juice in an electric blender or food processor and leave to stand for 15 minutes. Process to chop.

2 Add the honey, sugar, and all but 2 tablespoons of yoghurt. Process until mixed and velvety.

3 Place in 4 individual serving dishes. Divide the remaining yoghurt between the tops of the prune velvet and swirl through the mix.

4 Sprinkle with orange rind and serve.

NUTRITIONAL VALUES

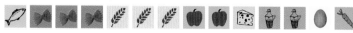

FRUIT COMPOTE WITH SMETANA

SERVES **4**

This can be eaten for breakfast or served up as a healthy dessert, too!

100 g dried prunes

100 g dried apricots

75 g dried pears

300 ml orange juice

150 ml water

strip of lemon rind, to garnish

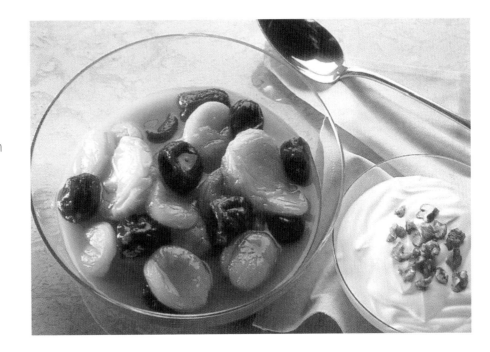

1 Place the prunes, apricots, pears, orange juice and water in a saucepan and bring to the boil.

2 Cover and simmer for 15 minutes. Leave to cool, covered.

3 Serve warm or chilled, topped with a spoonful of smetana and sprinkled with walnuts.

NUTRITIONAL VALUES

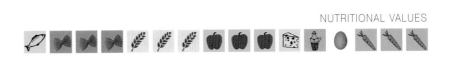

RAISIN BRAN CRUNCH

MAKES **1 kg**

A very tasty and crunchy breakfast cereal that can be served with either milk or low-fat yoghurt.

heaped 150 g raisins

525 g bran

170 g oatmeal

12 tbsp sesame seeds (preferably unroasted)

10 tbsp sunflower seeds (unroasted)

250 ml less 2 tbsp unsweetened orange juice

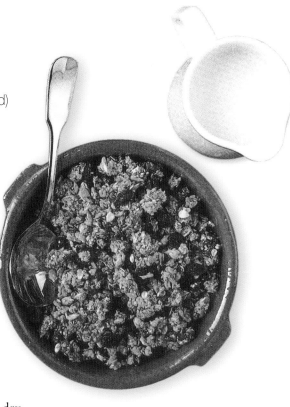

1 Mix the raisins, bran, oatmeal and both types of seeds in a large bowl, then stir in the orange juice.

2 Preheat the oven at 160°C/gas mark 3.

3 Lightly grease a large roasting pan. Stir the mixture thoroughly, then turn it into the pan – do not press it down. Bake for about 2 hours, turning and stirring occasionally, until well browned, crisp and dry.

4 Allow to cool in the pan, then break the mixture up into small lumps and store them in an airtight container.

5 Serve with milk.

NUTRITIONAL VALUES

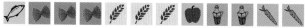

APRICOT YOGHURT CRUNCH

SERVES 4

A variation on a Scottish dish, the crunchy oatmeal, spicy yoghurt and lightly poached fruit make an attractive morning dish.

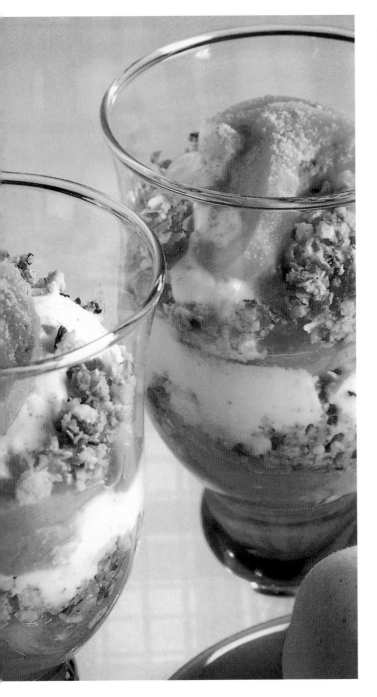

300 g apricots, pitted

3 tbsp honey

85 g oatmeal, toasted

1/2–1 tsp ground ginger

375 g low-fat plain yoghurt

1   Place the apricots in a pan with 170 ml water and 1 tablespoon of the honey. Cook for 5 minutes until softened and drain.

2   Mix the oatmeal and remaining honey in a bowl. Stir the ginger into the yoghurt. Alternatively layer the fruit, yoghurt and oatmeal mixtures into serving glasses. Chill and serve.

NUTRITIONAL VALUES

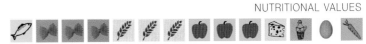

HASH-BROWN POTATOES WITH BAKED BEANS

These golden potato cakes are served with a spicy bean dish, and are perfect for mopping up the delicious juices. Make the bean dish in advance and keep in the refrigerator until morning. Simply heat the beans in a pan over gentle heat.

FOR THE BAKED BEANS

180 g dried harricot beans, soaked overnight

10 ml vegetable stock (see page 24)

1/2 tsp dried mustard

1 onion, chopped

2 tbsp dark molasses

140 g tomatoes, peeled and chopped

1 tbsp tomato purée

1 tbsp fresh basil, chopped

freshly ground black pepper

FOR THE POTATO CAKES

750 g potatoes, peeled and cubed

2 tbsp skimmed milk

1 onion, chopped

1 garlic clove, crushed

2 tsp olive oil

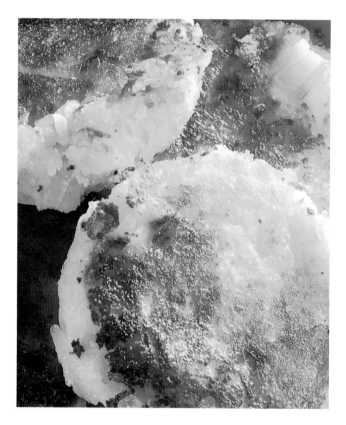

1 Drain the soaked beans and rinse well under cold water. Drain and put in a large saucepan with 450 ml of water. Bring the beans to the boil and boil rapidly for 10 minutes. Reduce the heat to a simmer, cover and cook for 1 hour or until the beans are cooked, topping up the water, if necessary. Drain the beans and return them to the pan. Stir in the vegetable stock, dried mustard, onion, molasses, tomatoes, tomato purée and basil. Season well and cook for 15 minutes or until the vegetables have cooked.

2 Make the potato cakes while the beans are cooking. Cook the potatoes in boiling water for 20 minutes or until just soft. Drain well and mash with the milk.

3 Add the onion and garlic, mixing well, and form into 12 equal-sized cakes. Brush a non-stick frying pan with the olive oil and warm over medium heat. Cook the potato cakes for 15–20 minutes, turning once, until golden brown. Serve piping hot with the baked beans.

NUTRITIONAL VALUES

LIGHT MEALS

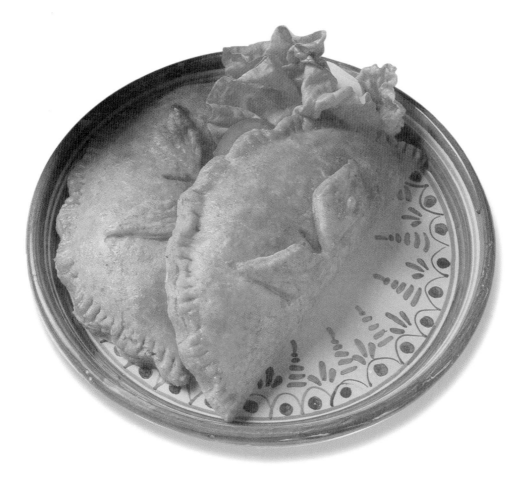

TAGLIATELLE WITH CHICKPEAS AND BASIL

SERVES **4**

Pasta and chickpeas with aromatic fresh basil make a wonderful combination of flavours.

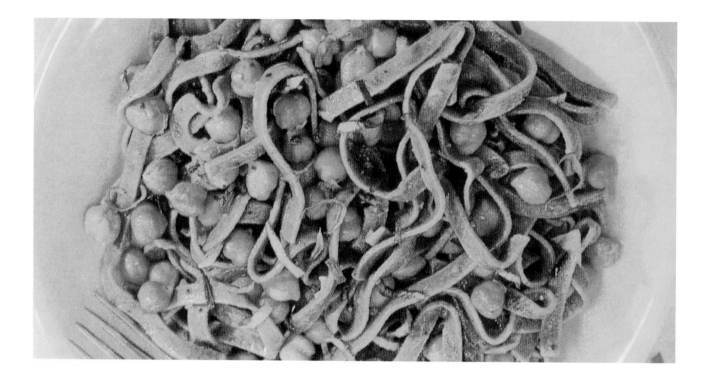

4 tbsp olive oil

1 garlic clove, crushed

6 tbsp chives, snipped

4 sage leaves, chopped

salt substitute (see page 12) and freshly ground
  black pepper

2 x 350 g can chickpeas, drained

450 g tagliatelle verdi

6 basil sprigs

1 Heat the olive oil, garlic, chives, sage, salt substitute and freshly ground black pepper with the chickpeas in a large saucepan for about 3 minutes. The idea is to heat the ingredients rather than to cook them.

2 Add the drained pasta and toss well. Leave the pan over the lowest heat setting while you use scissors to shred the basil sprigs over the pasta, discarding any tough stalk ends.

NUTRITIONAL VALUES

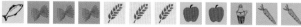

TAGLIATELLE WITH LENTIL SAUCE

SERVES **4**

This simple recipe is quick to make and ideal for lunch or supper.

350 g dried tagliatelle

dash of olive oil

2 tbsp butter

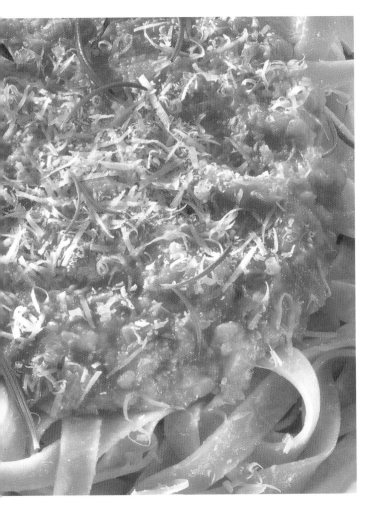

FOR THE SAUCE

200 g red lentils, washed and drained

3 tbsp tomato purée

salt substitute (see p 12) and freshly ground black
pepper

600 ml boiling water

sprigs of fresh rosemary, to garnish

freshly grated Parmesan cheese, to serve

1 Bring a large saucepan of water to the boil, and
add the tagliatelle with a dash of olive oil. Cook
for about 10 minutes, stirring occasionally, until
tender. Drain, and return to the saucepan. Add
the butter and stir. Cover and set aside, to keep
warm.

2 To make the lentil sauce, heat the olive oil in a
large saucepan and sauté the garlic and onion for
about 5 minutes, stirring occasionally, until
softened. Add the lentils, tomato purée, salt
substitute and ground black pepper, and stir in the
boiling water. Bring to the boil, then simmer for
about 20 minutes, stirring occasionally, until the
lentils have softened.

3 Reheat the tagliatelle gently for 2–3 minutes, if
necessary, then serve with the lentil sauce. Scatter
a few sprigs of fresh rosemary over the top, and
serve with freshly grated Parmesan cheese.

NUTRITIONAL VALUES

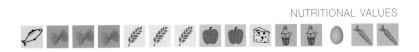

CARAMELIZED ONION TART

SERVES **6 – 8**

This is a sweet and delicious onion light meal, and it can also be served in smaller portions as a starter.

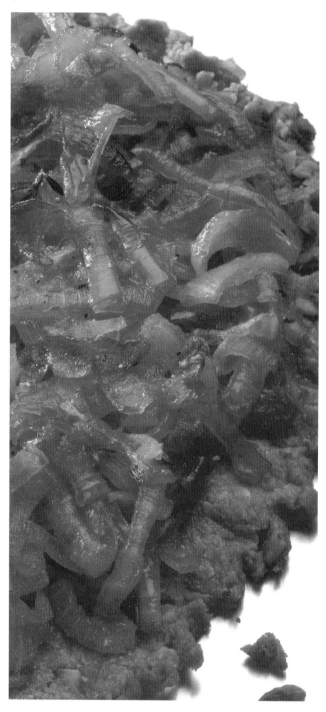

700 g onions, sliced

3 tbsp olive oil

6 small cloves garlic, peeled and left whole

3 bay leaves

salt substitute (see page 12) and freshly ground
black pepper

4–5 sprigs fresh thyme

BASE

40 g toasted hazelnuts or almonds, chopped

175 g wholemeal flour

$\frac{1}{2}$ tsp salt substitute (see page 12)

1 egg, beaten

50 ml olive oil

1 Cook the onions in the olive oil until they start to brown, then add the garlic, herbs and seasonings. Cook slowly for at least 1 hour, until softened and lightly browned.

2 Make the base by blending the dry ingredients together, then binding them with the egg and olive oil. Work into a dough, then roll out to a rough circle about 25 cm in diameter on a baking sheet. Chill for at least 45 minutes.

3 Preheat oven to 220°C/gas mark 7. Remove the bay leaves from the onion mixture; spread it over the nut base. Grind some black pepper over the onions, drizzle a little extra olive oil on top and bake for 25 minutes, until the base is lightly browned. Cool slightly before serving.

NUTRITIONAL VALUES

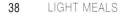

CHOLE

SERVES **8–10**

This recipe for soured chickpeas is full of fibre.

200 g chickpeas, washed

825 ml water

1 teabag

3 tbsp olive oil

225 g potatoes, boiled and diced into 1/2 in cubes

2 medium onions, finely chopped

1 clove garlic, crushed

2 tsp ground coriander

2 green chillies, chopped

1 1/2 tbsp amchoor

1/2 tsp chilli powder

175 ml water

1 1/2 tsp garam masala

1   Soak the chickpeas in the water with the teabag overnight.

2   Discard the teabag and place the chickpeas and the water in a saucepan and bring to boil. Cover and simmer for about 1 hour until tender. Drain.

3   Heat the oil in a saucepan over medium heat and fry the diced potatoes until lightly browned. Set aside.

4   In the remaining oil fry the onions until golden brown. Add the garlic and ginger and fry a further 2 minutes.

5   Add the chickpeas, coriander, green chillies, amchoor, chilli, and potatoes and stir fry for about 2 minutes until well mixed.

6   Add the water and cook for about 15 minutes. Sprinkle with garam masala. Serve hot with batora.

NUTRITIONAL VALUES

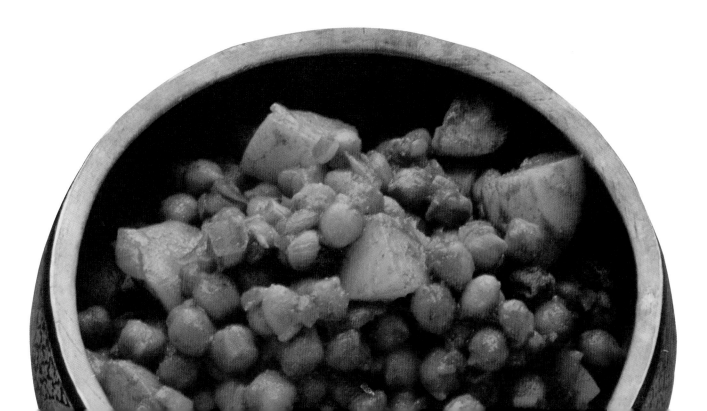

BEANS WITH MIXED GRAINS

SERVES **4**

*The combination of red and black beans and three different grains make this a
colourful dish with many different tastes and textures.*

50 g red kidney beans, soaked overnight

50 g black kidney beans, soaked overnight

short-grained rice measured to the 225 ml mark in
a measuring jug, washed and soaked

25 g millet

25 g pearl barley

1 Drain the beans, add to a saucepan of boiling
water, cover and bring to the boil. Boil for 10
minutes, then simmer for 1–1¹⁄₂ hours until just
tender; the time will depend on the beans. Drain
them, reserving the water.

2 Drain the rice. Put all the ingredients in a
saucepan, add 400 ml of the bean cooking water
and bring to the boil. Stir once, then cover and
turn the heat to very low. Cook for 20–30 minutes,
without removing the lid even once. Turn the heat
up as high as it will go for 30 seconds then turn it
off, or remove the pan from the heat. Leave,
without removing the lid at all, for 10–15 minutes
before serving.

NUTRITIONAL VALUES

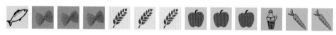

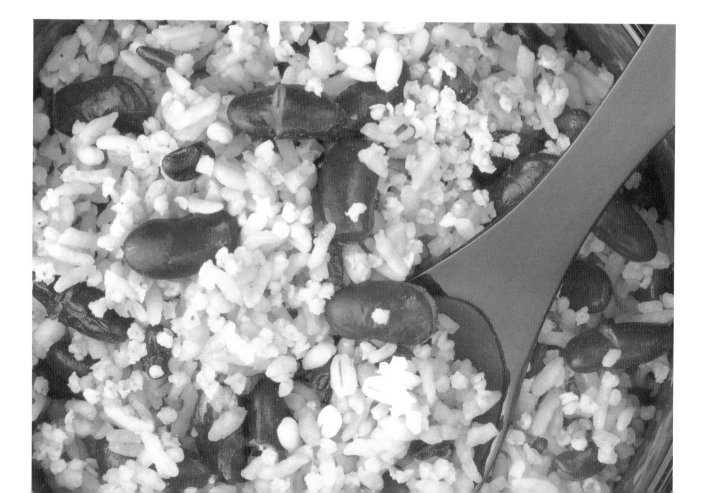

RAMEN WITH STIR-FRIED VEGETABLES

SERVES **4**

Ramen noodles topped with a blend of fresh and flash-fried vegetables – deliciously simple and simply delicious!

450 g ramen noodles or 400 g fresh or 350 g dried
   thin egg noodles

1.5 litres soy sauce stock

FOR THE TOPPING

2 tbsp olive oil

1 tbsp sesame oil

1 small onion, sliced

75 g mange tout, cut in half diagonally

2–3 small carrots, cut into long matchsticks

150 g bean sprouts

225 g Chinese cabbage, chopped

2 dried wood ear fungus or dried shiitake
   mushrooms, soaked in water, rinsed and
   chopped

freshly ground black pepper

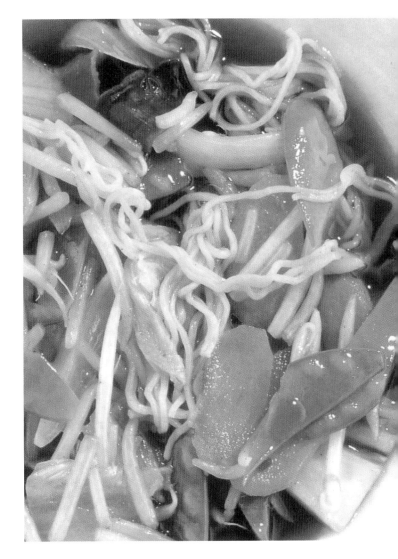

1   Make the topping. Heat the oils in a wok or frying pan until very hot. Stir-fry the onion, mange tout, and carrots for 2 minutes, then add the bean sprouts, Chinese cabbage, wood ear or shiitake mushrooms, and stir-fry for another 3–4 minutes. Season.

2   Boil plenty of water in a large pan and add the noodles. Cook for 3 minutes before draining well. Put the noodles into four bowls.

3   Heat the soy sauce stock. Pile the stir-fried vegetables onto the noodles and pour the stock over the top.

NUTRITIONAL VALUES

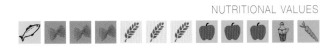

SPINACH QUICHE

A very traditional light meal, which can be adapted by using other vegetables. If you want to try something other than spinach, you could use leeks, mushrooms, onions or peppers as delicious alternatives.

175 g wholemeal pastry

FILLING

450 g spinach

salt substitute (see page 12) and freshly ground
   black pepper

1 spring onion, washed and chopped

2 eggs

4 tbsp low-fat cream

4 tbsp milk (for 22.5 cm flan ring only)

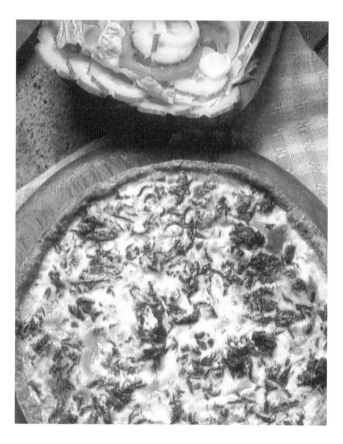

1 Make up the pastry and rest in the refrigerator for 15 minutes.

2 Line a 20 cm flan ring.

3 Fill with baking beans on waxed paper or crumpled foil and bake empty at 200°C/gas mark 6 for 15 minutes. Remove the beans and allow to cool slightly.

4 Cook the spinach for a few minutes to thaw. Drain well and squeeze out excess moisture. Arrange in the bottom of the flan ring, sprinkle with seasoning and chopped spring onion.

5 Mix the egg and low-fat cream with more seasoning and, if using the larger size flan, add 1 tablespoon of milk. Pour over the spinach and bake at 180°C/gas mark 4 until golden and set. This will take about 20 minutes.

6 Serve hot or cold with a crisp salad.

VARIATION

Onion and pepper quiche

Peel and slice thinly 2 onions. Seed and cut 1 red or green pepper into rings. Heat 25 g butter in a frying pan and cook the onions and pepper rings for 5 minutes, over a low heat to prevent browning. Arrange on the bottom of the flan ring and finish as for Spinach quiche.

NUTRITIONAL VALUES

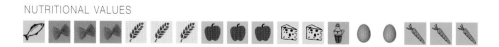

CUCUMBER TABBOULEH

SERVES **6**

A traditional tabbouleh is almost green in colour from the high proportion of herbs to cracked wheat. It is important to dry the wheat thoroughly or the finished salad will be soggy and unpalatable.

150 g fine cracked wheat or bulgur

425 ml boiling water

15 g parsley, chopped

15 g mint, chopped

2 tomatoes, deseeded and chopped

2 spring onion, trimmed and finely chopped

$^1/_2$ cucumber, diced

juice of 1 lemon

salt substitute (see page 12) and freshly ground
   black pepper

50 ml fruity olive oil

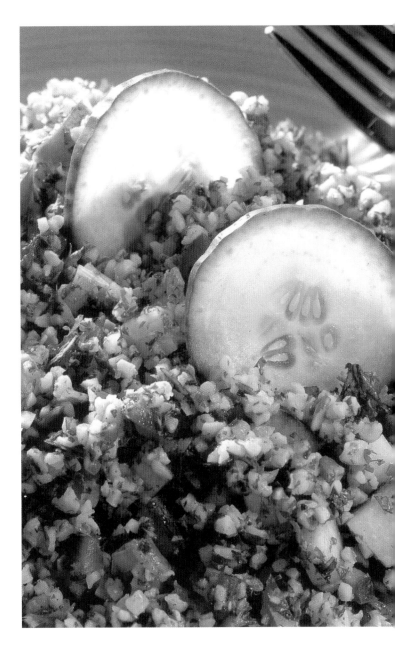

1 Allow the cracked wheat to soak in the boiling water for 30 minutes then drain, if necessary, and squeeze dry in a clean tea towel.

2 Place the wheat in a large bowl and add all the remaining ingredients, including seasonings to taste. Toss the salad well and serve at room temperature.

NUTRITIONAL VALUES

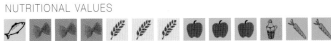

APRICOT, ALMOND AND TOMATO SALAD

SERVES **4 – 6**

Served with warm crusty wholemeal bread, this salad is a meal in itself.

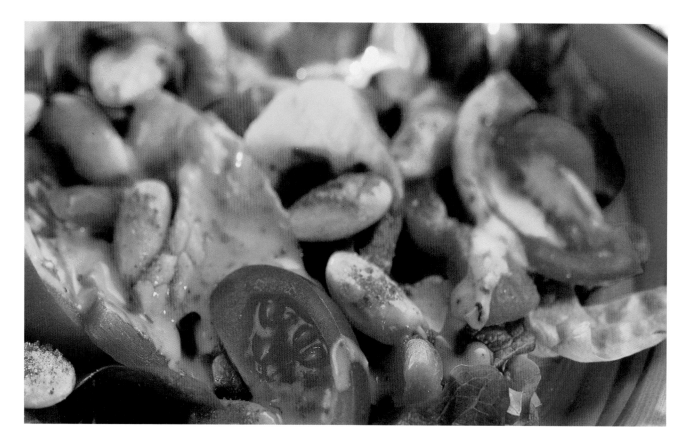

100 g blanched almonds

salt substitute (see page 12)

ground cayenne pepper

salad leaves

4 ripe tomatoes, cut into wedges

200 g dried apricots, roughly chopped

6 tbsp mustard-flavoured vinaigrette

parsley

1 Heat a frying pan, preferably non-stick, until evenly hot, then add the almonds. Cook over moderate heat until evenly browned on both sides (the almonds may be toasted if preferred). Dust some absorbent kitchen paper with salt substitute and cayenne pepper, then add the hot almonds and toss until well coated with the seasonings. Allow to cool, tossing from time to time.

2 Line a salad bowl with mixed leaves of your choice. Mix together the tomatoes, chopped apricots and deviled almonds and arrange them over the salad leaves. Spoon on the mustard vinaigrette and garnish with a sprig of parsley.

NUTRITIONAL VALUES

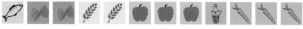

RICE AND ROASTED PEPPER SALAD

SERVES **4**

This salad has its origins in France, where leftover rice is dressed with vinaigrette and tossed with fresh vegetables such as peppers, olives and herbs.

250 g brown rice, preferably long-grain

4 to 5 cloves garlic, chopped

¼ onion, chopped

1 medium bottle green pimiento-stuffed olives, halved

1 red pepper, roasted, peeled and chopped

1 to 3 mild to medium green chillies, roasted, peeled and chopped

½–1 tsp French mustard, preferably Dijon

generous pinch each: turmeric and curry powder

1 tbsp mixed fresh herbs: sage, mint, coriander, and oregano, or to taste

salt substitute (see page 12) and freshly ground black pepper

dash of Tabasco or hot sauce

1 ripe tomato, diced, including the juices

3–4 tbsp extra-virgin olive oil

1 tbsp white wine vinegar

1 tsp balsamic vinegar

1 tbsp fresh parsley, chopped

NUTRITIONAL VALUES

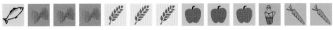

1 Cook the rice in 250 ml water until it is tender but still firm to the bite, then fork to separate. If using freshly made rice add the rest of the ingredients and leave to cool. Season to taste before serving.

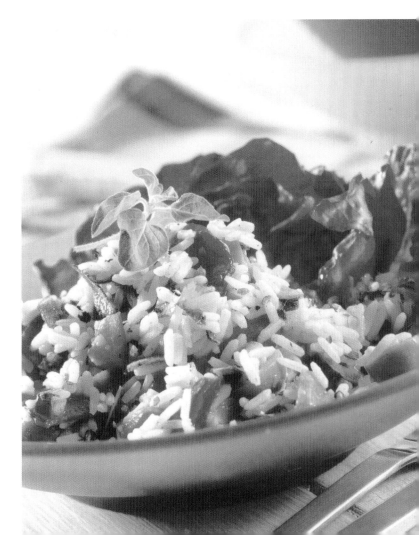

MIXED BEAN SALAD

SERVES **4**

A good bean salad needs a tangy dressing to succeed. The garlic and lemon-based dressing provides a tasty complement to the texture of the salad.

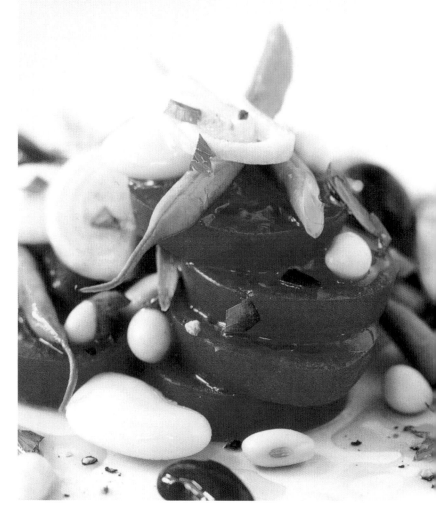

200 g green beans, trimmed and halved

6 tbsp tinned soya beans

4 tbsp tinned butter beans

4 tbsp tinned red kidney beans

1 shallot, sliced

FOR THE DRESSING

$\frac{1}{2}$ clove garlic, finely chopped

2 tbsp freshly squeezed lemon juice

4 tbsp extra-virgin olive oil

salt substitute (see page 12) and freshly
    ground black pepper

1 tbsp fresh parsley, chopped

2 medium tomatoes, sliced for decoration

black olives for garnishing

1 Cook the green beans in a pan of boiling water for 3–4 minutes and drain. Rinse the beans well.

2 Put all the beans and the shallot in a bowl, sprinkle with salt substitute and pepper and mix well.

3 Combine the garlic, lemon juice, oil and parsley in a jar and shake well.

4 Lay the sliced tomato on a serving dish, pile the bean mixture in the centre, sprinkle with dressing and garnish with olives.

NUTRITIONAL VALUES

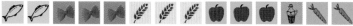

ONION AND SAFFRON RISOTTO

SERVES **4**

The temptation with risotto is to add too many flavouring ingredients. Resist at all costs! Just the onion and saffron are a perfect combination, particularly when garnished with the fried garlic.

1.5 litres vegetable stock (see page 24)

2 tbsp olive oil

1 tbsp butter

1 large onion and 2 red onions, chopped

few strands saffron

225 g arborio rice

olive oil to deep-fry

2 large cloves garlic, sliced

salt substitute (see page 12) and freshly ground black pepper

1 Set the vegetable stock to the boil, then heat the oil and butter together in a large frying pan, add the chopped onions, and cook slowly for 6–8 minutes, until softened but not browned. Add the saffron to the boiling stock.

2 Stir the rice into the frying pan and coat it in the onion juices, then add about one-third of the stock. Simmer until absorbed, stirring from time to time, then add half the remaining stock. Continue until all the stock has been absorbed into the risotto, giving a moist, creamy consistency – add a little more stock if necessary.

3 Meanwhile, heat about 2.5 cm of olive oil in a small pan, add the garlic slices and fry until golden brown. Drain on paper towels – keep the olive oil to add to mashed potatoes or to use for frying.

4 Season the risotto to taste and serve hot, garnished with the fried garlic.

NUTRITIONAL VALUES

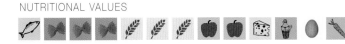

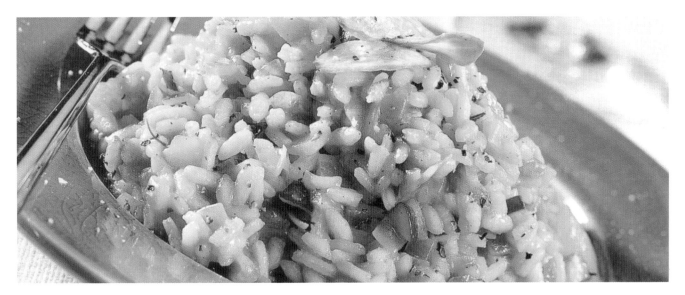

REFRIED KIDNEY BEANS

The more often you refry the beans, the better they taste!

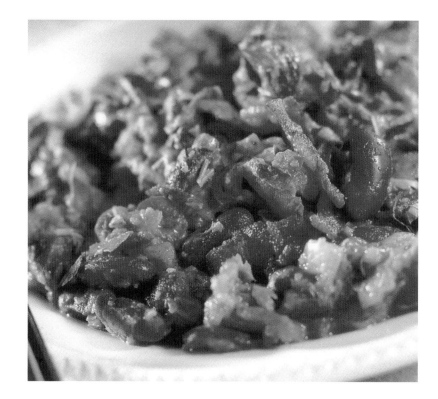

450 g can kidney beans

1 red chilli, deseeded and chopped

1 medium onion, finely chopped

2 tsp garlic, crushed

1 tsp paprika

freshly ground black pepper

1.25 litres water

6 slices good bacon, without the rind

2 tbsp olive oil

parsley, to serve

1 Place the first 7 ingredients in a pan, bring to the boil and simmer for 40 minutes.

2 Place one-quarter of the total in a food processor and purée. Remix the puréed beans with the whole beans.

3 Chop the bacon and place in boiling water for 10 minutes to remove the saltiness. Remove from the water and drain.

4 Heat the butter in a frying pan and fry the bacon. Add the beans, little by little, and mash with the back of a spoon. Season well.

5 The beans should go into a thick purée. Season, sprinkle with parsley and serve. The more often you refry the beans, the better they taste.

NUTRITIONAL VALUES

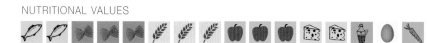

BRAISED SOYA BEANS

SERVES **4**

The humble soya bean is the most widely used ingredient in Japanese cuisine, forming the basis for soy sauce, tofu and miso. Soya beans are rich in nutrients and fibre and are regarded in Japan as 'meat from the earth'.

3 dried shiitake mushrooms

7.5 cm dried kelp, wiped with a damp cloth

420 g tinned soya beans, drained

50 g carrots, peeled and diced

2 tbsp granulated sugar

1½ tbsp soy sauce

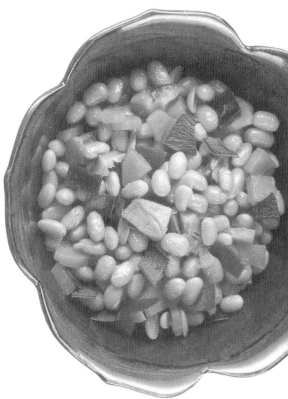

1 Soak the shiitake mushrooms and kelp in 200 ml of water for 30 minutes. Reserve the water. Dice the shiitake mushrooms and kelp into small pieces.

2 Put the kelp, mushrooms, and reserved water into a pan. Add the soya beans, carrot, an extra 100 ml of fresh water and the sugar. Bring to the boil and cook, uncovered, for 15 minutes.

3 Add the soy sauce and simmer for a further 10 minutes. Serve as a side dish. Any leftovers can be stored in a fridge for up to a week.

NUTRITIONAL VALUES

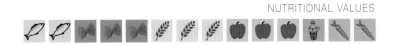

ONION AND CHILLI TABBOULEH

SERVES **6**

Tabbouleh, a salad of bulgur wheat, is usually flavoured with herbs. In this version onions and chillies can be used for a little more spice.

150 g fine bulgur

450 ml boiling water

6 spring onions, finely chopped

1 red and 1 green chilli, finely chopped

½ cucumber, finely diced

250 ml watercress, chopped

juice of ½ lemon

freshly ground black pepper

4 tbsp green olive oil

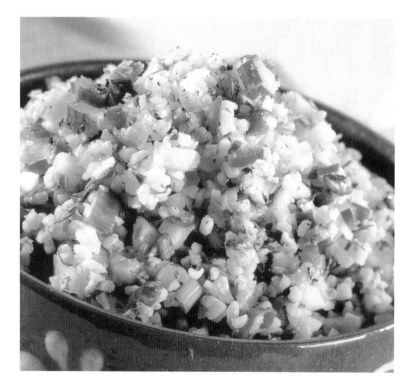

1   Place the bulgur in a bowl, pour over the boiling water and allow to stand for 30 minutes. Drain, then squeeze dry through a fine sieve or in a clean dish towel.

2   Turn the bulgar into a large bowl and mix in all the remaining ingredients. Mix well, then serve at room temperature.

NUTRITIONAL VALUES

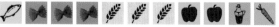

POTATO PIE

SERVES **6**

This pie can also be served as a main course, along with a green salad garnished with a few finely chopped shallots.

4 shallots

750 g potatoes

salt substitute (see page 12) and freshly ground
  black pepper

pinch of nutmeg

1 sheet ready-rolled pastry dough

250 ml low-fat crème fraîche

200 g Conté, Emmenthal or Gruyère cheese,
  grated

1 sheet ready-rolled puff pastry

1 medium egg yolk

1 Preheat the oven to 190°C/gas mark 5.

2 Peel and thinly slice the shallots. Peel, wash and dry the potatoes. Cut them into thin slices. In a bowl, mix together the potatoes and shallots. Add the seasoning and nutmeg, and mix thoroughly.

3 Place the pastry dough in a 25 cm round buttered pie pan, allowing it to overlap the dish slightly.

4 Place half of the potatoes and shallots on the pie base. Spread them out, then coat with half of the low-fat crème fraîche, followed by half of the grated cheese. Repeat to make a second layer.

5 Unroll the puff pastry and place over the top of the dish, cutting off the excess. Seal the edges with the overlapping pastry dough, pinching regularly between your fingers, moistened with cold water. Using a sharp knife, make a slit in the middle and insert a strip of foil wound around itself several times as a funnel. This will enable the steam to escape during cooking. Score the surface of the puff pastry using a sharp knife.

6 Dilute the egg yolk with a little water to make a glaze. With a pastry brush, generously coat the top of the pie. Place in the oven for 1 hour, covering with foil to prevent over-browning. Serve very hot.

NUTRITIONAL VALUES

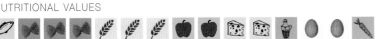

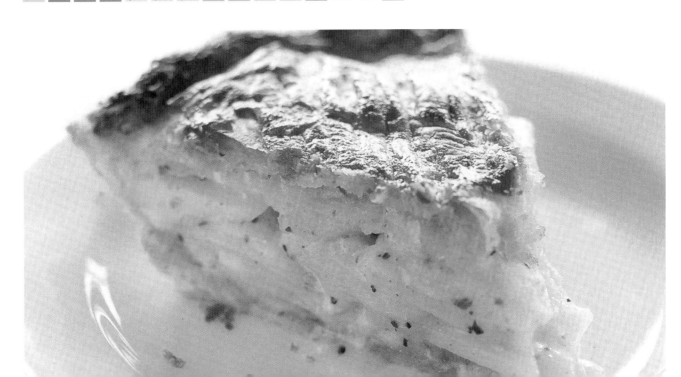

WHEAT BERRY WALDORF SALAD

This salad is served lightly seasoned with salt substitute and pepper, and garnished with roasted walnuts if required.

4 oz wheat berries (wholegrain, hard wheat)

1³/₄ pt water

1 tsp salt substitute (see page 12)

1 McIntosh apple, diced

1 Granny Smith apple, diced

1³/₄ pt water mixed with 2 tbsp lemon juice

1 small stalk celery, diced

2 oz dried sour cherries

2 oz saltanas

3 tbsp fresh mint, chopped

4 spring onions, thinly sliced

3 tbsp seasoned rice wine vinegar

3 tbsp fresh orange juice

1 tsp orange rind, grated

¹/₂ tsp white pepper

2 tbsp walnuts, roasted and chopped

NUTRITIONAL VALUES

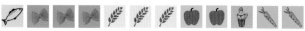

1 In a saucepan bring the water and lemon juice to the boil and add the wheat berries. Reduce the heat and simmer, covered, for 1¹/₂ hours or until tender. Drain the wheat berries in a colander and cool to room temperature. Place the apples in the lemon water and set aside. Combine the celery, cherries, sultanas, mint and spring onions in a large bowl.

2 In another bowl combine the vinegar, orange juice and orange rind. Drain the apples and add them to the celery mixture. Add the cooled wheat berries. Pour the orange juice mixture over the wheat berries and toss until well blended. Season with salt substitute and pepper and garnish with roasted walnuts.

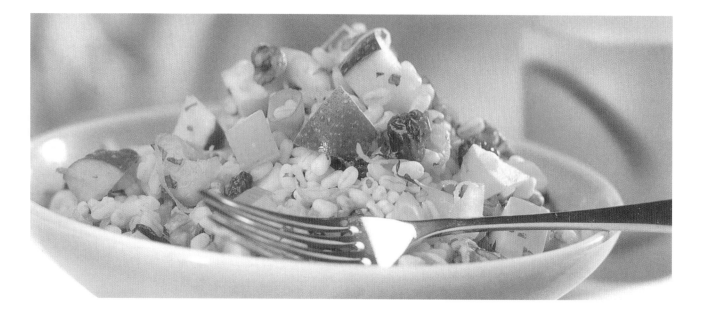

PASTA SALAD

SERVES **1 2**

Pasta salad makes an excellent buffet dish but, for everyday eating, it is a meal in itself. Some salads are dressed in vinaigrette, but you could alternatively add strained cottage cheese or plain yoghurt to a little low-fat mayonnaise.

225 g wholemeal pasta shapes of your choice

1 red pepper, deseeded and diced

125 g button mushrooms, halved

¹/₂ cucumber, diced

175 g sweetcorn

6 spring onions, finely sliced

426 g can red kidney beans, drained and rinsed

100 g diced Swiss cheese

salt substitute (see page 12) and freshly ground
    black pepper

salad leaves for serving

DRESSING

350 g strained cottage cheese or plain yoghurt

225 g low-fat mayonnaise

salt substitute (see page 12) and freshly ground
    black pepper

2–3 cloves garlic, crushed

15 g freshly chives, chopped

1 Bring a large pan of water to the boil and add the pasta. Return to the boil, then simmer as directed until just tender. Drain the pasta and rinse it in cold water, then let cool completely.

2 Mix all the prepared vegetables together and season lightly with salt substitute and pepper. Blend all the ingredients for the dressing and season to taste.

3 Place the pasta in a large bowl, then top with the vegetables. Spoon on the dressing. If the salad is prepared in advance, try leaving it in layers and tossing at the last minute. If it is to be served immediately, however, toss all the ingredients together then transfer the salad to a large platter, lined with greens.

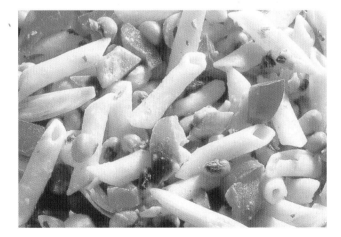

NUTRITIONAL VALUES

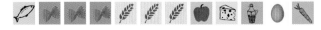

RAVIOLI IN TOMATO DRESSING

SERVES **4**

A cold pasta dish served in a tangy tomato sauce, ideal to serve on a hot sunny day for lunch.

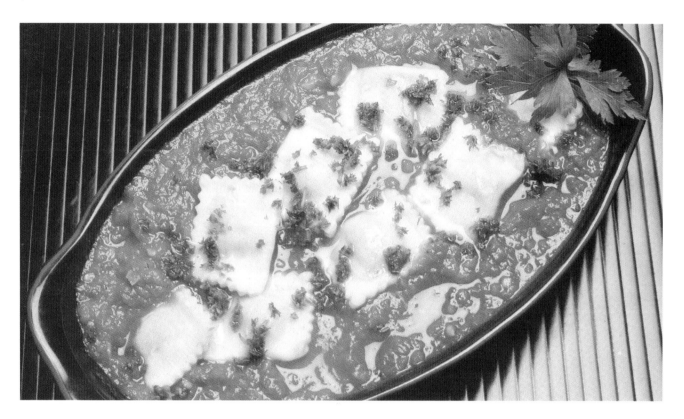

225 g cooked ravioli

TOMATO DRESSING

450 g tomatoes, skinned and chopped

1 tbsp fresh basil leaves or parsley

1 tsp lemon juice

salt substitute (see page 12) and freshly ground
   black pepper

4 tbsp olive oil

1 clove garlic, crushed

1 Make up the dressing in a jar with a screw-top as can be done for French dressing.

2 Chop the basil or parsley finely and add all ingredients to the jar, shake vigorously and leave to stand for at least half an hour in the refrigerator before using.

3 Shake well and coat the cooked cold ravioli.

NUTRITIONAL VALUES

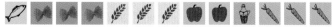

SWISS GREEN BEAN PIZZA

MAKES **30 cm DEEP PAN PIZZA**

Try this pizza when green beans are in season, especially if they come from your own garden. It turns an ordinary vegetable into a treat.

1 batch Wholemeal Pizza Dough (see below)

450 g fresh green beans

2 tbsp olive oil

50 g sliced almonds

100 g Swiss cheese, grated

1   Preheat the oven to 250°C/gas mark 9.

2   Wash and snip off the ends of the green beans. Steam them for 5–7 minutes, until crisp-tender. Then arrange the beans on the pizza dough. Sprinkle the olive oil over the beans. Next, sprinkle on the sliced almonds and top with the Swiss cheese. Bake for 10 minutes.

WHOLEMEAL PIZZA DOUGH

1 packet active dry yeast

250 ml warm water

300 g unbleached white flour

2 tbsp olive oil

½ tsp salt substitute (see page 12)

250 g wholemeal flour

1   In a large bowl, combine the yeast, warm water and white flour. Mix well to blend. Add the oil, salt substitute and wholemeal flour and stir until the dough sticks together. Place the dough on a lightly floured surface. Dust your hands with flour and then knead the dough until it is smooth and elastic, about 5 minutes. If the dough gets sticky, sprinkle it with a little more flour.

2   Roll the dough into a ball and place it in a lightly oiled bowl. Cover the bowl with a dish cloth and set in a warm, but not hot, place to rise until doubled in volume, about one hour.

3   When the dough has risen, roll it into a ball to make one deep pan pizza or divide it in two balls to make two thin-crust 30 cm pizzas. Before rolling out and topping the pizza, allow the dough to rest for 20 minutes.

4   When ready to bake, place dough in centre of lightly oiled pan. Roll outwards towards the edges with the palm of your hand until the dough fills the pan evenly.

NUTRITIONAL VALUES

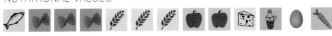

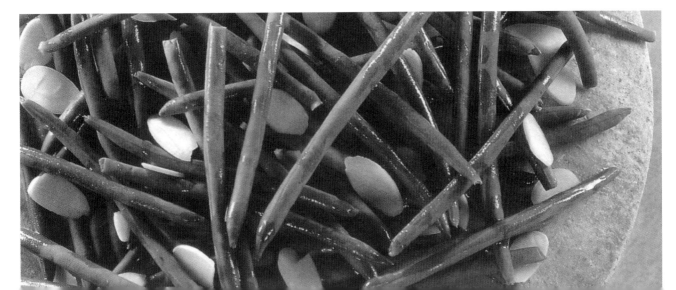

CHILLI BEAN RISOTTO

SERVES **4**

Packed full of the flavours of Mexico, this tasty risotto makes a tasty light meal for four people.

1.1 litres vegetable stock (see page 24)

2 tbsp olive oil

1 large onion, finely chopped

1 garlic clove, crushed

1 green chilli, deseeded and finely chopped

2 green peppers, deseeded and diced

400 g arborio rice

1 tsp ground cumin

1 tsp ground coriander

1 tsp chilli powder

freshly ground black pepper

400 g can kidney beans, drained and rinsed

350 g can sweetcorn, drained and rinsed

4 medium tomatoes, peeled, deseeded and
    chopped

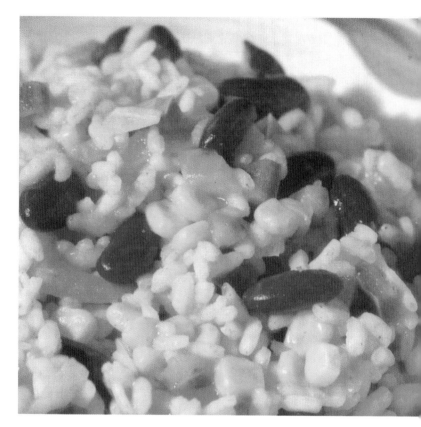

1   Pour the stock into a saucepan and bring to the boil. Reduce the heat to a gentle simmer.

2   Meanwhile, heat the oil in a large saucepan and gently fry the onion, garlic, chilli and green peppers for 4–5 minutes until softened, but not browned. Stir in the rice and cook, stirring, for 2 minutes until the rice is coated in the vegetable mixture.

3   Add a ladleful of stock and cook gently, stirring, until absorbed. Continue adding the stock ladle-by-ladle until half the stock is used. Stir in the spices, seasoning and kidney beans.

4   Continue adding the stock until the risotto becomes thick, but not sticky. This will take about 25 minutes and shouldn't be hurried.

5   Stir in the sweetcorn and tomatoes. Mix well, adjust seasoning if necessary, and serve.

NUTRITIONAL VALUES

NTAKOS

SERVES **4**

This utterly refreshing salad-sandwich, pronounced 'Dakos', hails from the island of Crete, and is healthy, delicious and rich in vitamins and fibre. It also wonderfully shows off the fresh flavours of the vegetables and the olive oil.

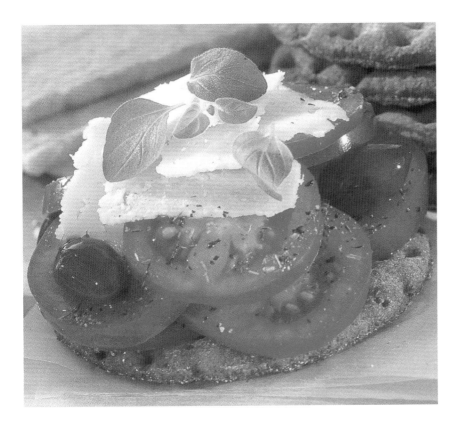

4 paximadia or other wholemeal crackers

12 or more ripe, sweet, juicy tomatoes

sprinkle of oregano

approximately 3 dozen black Greek or other Mediterranean olives, stoned and cut into pieces

175–225 g or sokefalotiri or pecorino cheese, thinly sliced or shaved

75–125 ml olive oil (preferably Greek), or as needed

1 Arrange the paximadia on a platter or on plates. Layer with the tomatoes, oregano, olives and cheese, and drizzle with olive oil.

2 Leave to marinate for at least four hours at room temperature, then serve.

NUTRITIONAL VALUES

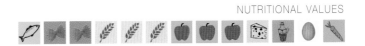

BLACK BEAN AND MANY-PEPPER CHILLI

SERVES **6**

This black bean chilli, rich with sweet and spicy peppers, is delicious on its own in a bowl topped with low-fat sour cream, crisp tortilla chips, chopped onions and grated cheese. It is also good as a sauce for most barbecued dishes and, thinned with stock, it makes a hearty soup.

400 g black beans

1.5 litres water

600 ml vegetable stock (see page 24)

2 dried mild red chillies, sliced

2 tbsp olive oil

2 red peppers, diced

1/2 green and yellow pepper, diced

1 onion, chopped

1/2 carrot, diced

8 cloves garlic, chopped

2 tsp mild chilli powder

1 tbsp cumin

1 tsp oregano

1 tbsp paprika

400 g tomatoes, chopped

1 red or green chilli, such as Anaheim, chopped

50–75 ml fresh coriander, chopped

1 Put the beans and water in a saucepan and bring to the boil. Reduce the heat and cook until the beans are nearly tender, then add the stock and dried chillies, and continue to cook, adding more liquid if needed.

2 Pour the olive oil into a frying pan and sauté the peppers, onion, carrot and half the garlic, until softened. Sprinkle with chilli powder, cumin, oregano and paprika, and add the tomatoes. Cook for a few moments, then add to the simmering and almost-tender beans along with the remaining garlic and half the coriander.

3 Continue to cook until the beans are very tender and the sauce is rich and dark. Add the fresh chilli to taste. Serve sprinkled with the remaining coriander.

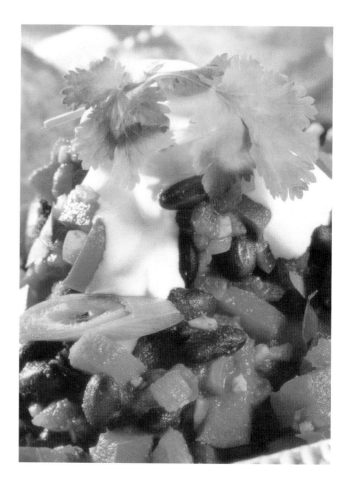

NUTRITIONAL VALUES

WHOLEMEAL PASTIES

SERVES **4**

These pasties are wholesome and high in fibre, and are ideal for putting in your lunch box or taking on a picnic.

225 g wholemeal pastry

1 large potato, peeled

2 carrots, scraped and diced

1 onion, peeled and diced

225 g chuck steak, trimmed

$^{1}/_{2}$ tsp Worcester sauce

freshly ground black pepper

$^{1}/_{2}$ tsp mixed herbs

$^{1}/_{2}$ pt beef stock

beaten egg (optional)

1 Make up the pastry and leave to rest in the refrigerator.

2 Dice the potato and mix with the diced carrots and chopped onion.

3 Cut the meat into 1.25 cm cubes. Put into a saucepan with the Worcester sauce, seasoning, herbs and stock. Turn on a low heat.

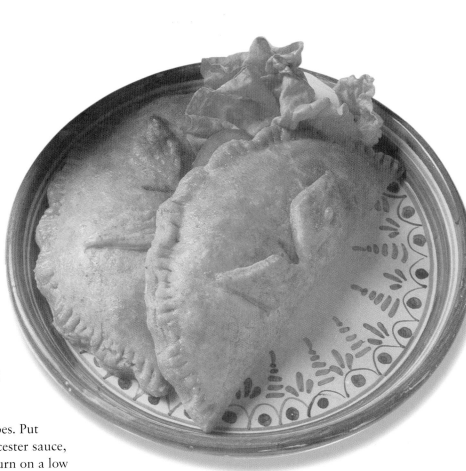

4 Add the vegetables and stir well until the mixture comes to the boil. Lower the heat and simmer for 30 minutes. Allow mixture to cool.

5 Divide the pastry into two and roll out half at a time to 0.5 cm thick. Cut two 15- to 17-cm rounds with a plate or flan ring.

6 Divide the meat mixture into four and place each portion in the centre of a ring of pastry. Wet the edges with a pastry brush dipped in cold water, fold the pastry rings in half. Crimp the edges and mark three small slits on each side with a sharp knife. If liked, brush with a little beaten egg to glaze.

7 Cook for 20 minutes at 200°C/gas mark 6, reduce the oven heat to 160°C/gas mark 3 and continue cooking for a further 15 minutes.

NUTRITIONAL VALUES

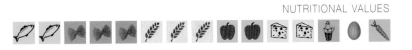

TUNA-STUFFED POTATOES

Especially good as a light meal for lunch, these stuffed potatoes also make a good accompaniment to a main course.

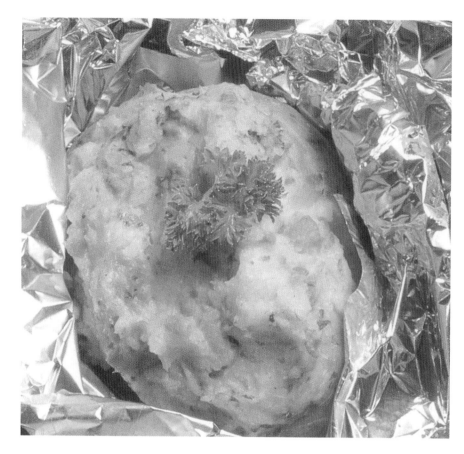

4 large potatoes, scrubbed

4 tomatoes, skinned and
chopped

4 spring onions, washed and
chopped

4 tbsp low-fat sour cream

freshly ground black pepper

200 g can tuna fish, in oil

1 Make a cross on the potato skins and bake for 1 hour at 180°C/gas mark 4 or until cooked.

2 Halve the potatoes and scoop out the cooked potato, retaining the skins.

3 Mix all ingredients together, season well and arrange in the potato skins.

4 Reheat before serving.

NUTRITIONAL VALUES

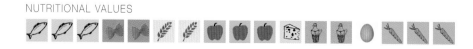

STARTERS

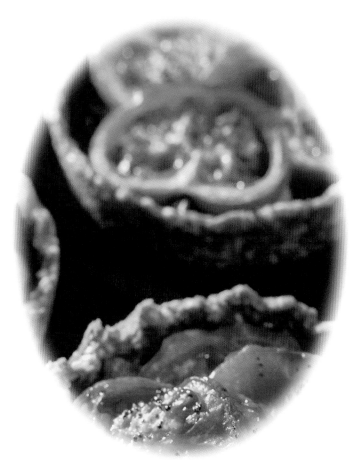

MIXED BEANS AND PASTA SOUP

SERVES **4**

A healthy, high-fibre soup with a Mediterranean flavour that is equally delicious served hot or chilled.

2 tbsp extra-virgin olive oil

1 medium onion, chopped

2 cloves garlic, chopped

1 courgette, chopped

1/2 tsp chilli powder

1 tsp ground coriander

4 tbsp tinned or frozen soya beans

4 tbsp tinned flageolet beans

1 litre vegetable (see page 24) or chicken
   stock (see page 25)

freshly ground black pepper

1 tomato, peeled and chopped

25 g small pasta shapes

coriander leaves

basil leaves, for garnish

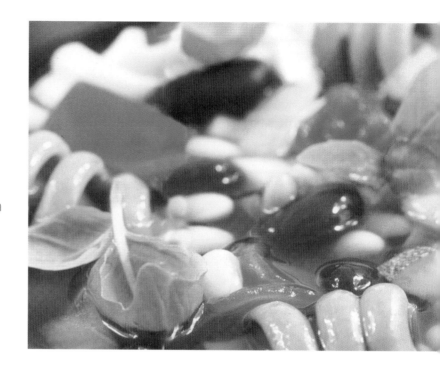

1   Heat the oil in a saucepan. Add the onion, garlic and courgette, and fry for 3 minutes or until softened.

2   Add the chilli powder, coriander, beans and stock. Season with pepper, then simmer for 30 minutes, covered.
Add the tomato, pasta and coriander leaves, and simmer for a further 10 minutes.
Garnish with the basil leaves.

NUTRITIONAL VALUES

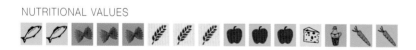

LENTIL SOUP

SERVES **4**

This is one of my favourite winter soups, and it is both nourishing and satisfying. The addition of cumin is an Anatolian variation that gives a distinctive taste.

2 tbsp olive oil

1 small onion, chopped

1 carrot, diced

825 ml chicken stock (see page 25)

150 g green lentils

1 tsp ground cumin

freshly ground black pepper

chopped fresh parsley, to garnish (optional)

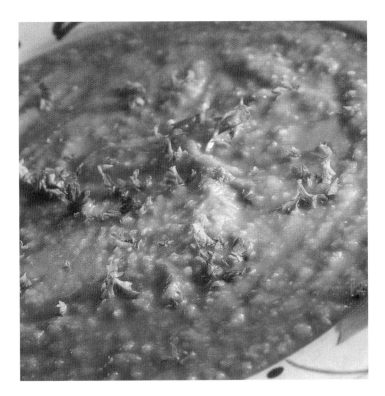

1 Heat the oil and fry the onion until soft. Add the carrot and cook for 1 minute.

2 Pour in the chicken stock and add the lentils. Bring to a boil over medium heat and stir in the cumin. Simmer for 20 minutes. Pass soup through a metal sieve or purée in a blender or food processor.

3 Return to the pan, reheat, taste and adjust the seasoning, and serve with parsley scattered over, if using.

NUTRITIONAL VALUES

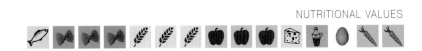

RICE AND PEAS

SERVES **4**

The real point of this extraordinary simple dish is the spiky flavour of fresh peas – so cook it only when the season is right. The texture, incidentally, is midway between soup and risotto, and requires a spoon.

2 tbsp olive oil

3 tbsp olive oil

1 small onion

900 g fresh peas, shelled

1 bouillon cube

225 g arborio rice

2 tbsp fresh parsley, finely chopped

85 g Parmesan, freshly grated

freshly ground black pepper, to taste

1 Heat the oil over a low heat.

2 Finely chop the onion and soften it in the oil. Add the peas and cook them for a further 2 minutes.

3 Crumble in the bouillon cube and add 750 ml of water. Bring the mixture to the boil.

4 As the water boils, add the parsley and the rice. Cook for about 15 minutes until the rice has softened but remains firm.

5 Whisk in the grated Parmesan, season with pepper and finish with a generous twist or three of black pepper.

NUTRITIONAL VALUES

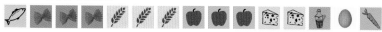

SMOKED CHICKEN AND LENTIL SOUP

SERVES **4**

A delicious and tasty wholesome soup to serve as a starter or a hot snack.

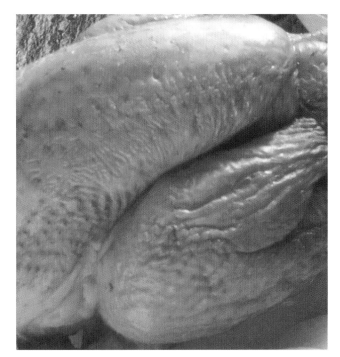

2 tbsp olive oil

2 leeks, split and thinly sliced

2 carrots, finely chopped

1 large onion, finely chopped

1 clove garlic, crushed

150 g dried lentils (preferably Puy)

450 ml water

bouquet garni (thyme sprigs, celery leaves, sage,
   and bay leaf)

1 litre chicken stock (see page 25)

200 g cubed smoked chicken

freshly ground black pepper

1 Heat the oil in a large saucepan or stockpot over medium heat. Add the leeks, carrots, onion and garlic, and cook for 4–5 minutes until slightly softened, stirring frequently.

2 Rinse and drain the lentils, and check for any small stones. Add to the vegetables with the water and bouquet garni. Bring to the boil, reduce the heat to medium-low and simmer for about 30 minutes, or until the lentils are just tender.

3 Add the chicken, season to taste with pepper, and continue cooking for 15 minutes. Remove the bouquet garni and ladle into a warm tureen or bowls.

NUTRITIONAL VALUES

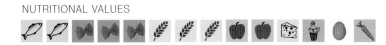

SPICY BLACK BEAN SOUP

SERVES **4 – 6**

This soup is served with a spoonful of low-fat sour cream and garnished with finely chopped spring onions and coriander.

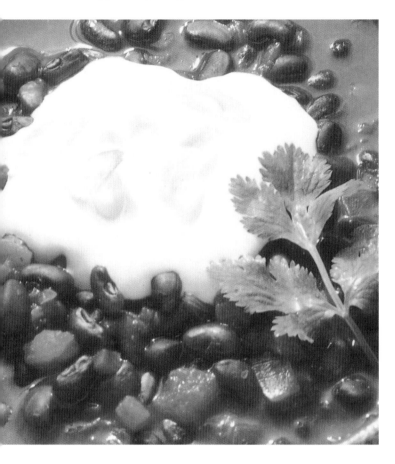

450 g black beans

1 tbsp olive oil

2 red onions, finely chopped

4 garlic cloves, crushed

5 tbsp brandy

2 litres water

bouquet garni (bay leaf, thyme, and marjoram
sprigs, coriander and parsley stems and 2–3
strips orange zest)

$^1\!/_2$ tsp cumin seeds

$^1\!/_4$ tsp dried oregano

3–4 roasted ancho chilli peppers, deseeded and
chopped, or $^3\!/_4$ tsp dried chillies, crushed

1 tbsp tomato purée

3 tomatoes, peeled, deseeded and chopped

salt substitute (see page 12) and freshly ground
black pepper

6 tbsp low-fat sour cream

3–4 spring onions, finely chopped

coriander leaves, for garnishing

1 Pick over the beans to remove any small stones. Cover with cold water and leave to soak for 6 hours or overnight.

2 Drain the beans, put into a saucepan with cold water to cover and set over high heat. Bring to the boil and boil for 10 minutes. Drain and rinse well.

3 Heat the oil in a large, heavy saucepan over medium–high heat, add the onions and cook until they are just softened, 3–4 minutes, stirring frequently. Add the garlic and continue cooking for 2 minutes. Add the brandy, water, bouquet garni, cumin seeds, oregano, and chillies. When the mixture begins to bubble, stir in the tomato purée, reduce the heat to low and simmer gently, partially covered, for 1$^1\!/_2$–2$^1\!/_2$ hours until the beans are tender, stirring occasionally. Remove and discard the bouquet garni and season with pepper, if you wish.

4 Ladle the soup into a warm tureen or bowls and top with a dollop of low-fat sour cream. Sprinkle with the spring onions and garnish with coriander.

NUTRITIONAL VALUES

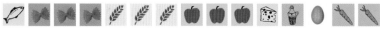

PROVENÇAL VEGETABLE SOUP

SERVES **6**

Served with a swirl of basil purée, this makes a very filling starter!

275 g fresh shelled fava, coco, or cranberry beans,
   or 175 g dried beans, soaked overnight

1/4 tsp dried herbes de Provence

2 cloves garlic, crushed

1 tbsp olive oil

1 medium onion, finely chopped

1 large leek, split and finely sliced

1 celery stick, finely sliced

2 thin carrots, finely diced

2 small potatoes, finely diced

125 g thin green beans

1.25 litres water

salt substitute (see page 12) and freshly ground
   black pepper

150 g shelled peas, fresh or frozen

2 small courgette, quartered lengthways and finely
   sliced

3 medium tomatoes, peeled, deseeded and finely
   chopped

a handful of spinach leaves, cut in thin ribbons

BASIL PURÉE

1 large or 2 small cloves garlic, very finely chopped

50 g (packed) basil leaves

4 tbsp freshly grated Parmesan cheese

4 tbsp extra-virgin olive oil

1 To make the basil purée, put the garlic, basil and cheese in a food processor fitted with a steel blade and process until thoroughly puréed, scraping down the sides once. With the machine running, slowly pour the olive oil through the feed tube. Alternatively, pound the garlic, basil and cheese in a pestle and mortar, then slowly stir in the oil.

2 Put the fresh or soaked beans in a large saucepan with the dried herbs and 1 of the garlic cloves, and add water to cover by 2.5 cm. Bring to the boil, reduce the heat and simmer over medium-low heat until the beans are cooked, about 20 minutes for fresh beans, or about 1 hour for dried beans. Set aside in the cooking liquid.

3 Heat the olive oil in a large saucepan over medium-low heat. Add the onion and leek, and cook for 5 minutes, stirring occasionally, until the onion softens. Add the celery, carrots and the remaining garlic, and cook covered for another 10 minutes, stirring frequently.

4 Add the potatoes, green beans and water. Season lightly with pepper. Bring to the boil, reduce the heat to low and simmer, covered, for 10 minutes.

5 Add the peas, courgette and tomatoes. Add the cooked broad beans with the cooking liquid and simmer for 25–30 minutes, or until all the vegetables are tender. Taste for seasoning. Add the spinach and simmer for 5 minutes longer. Ladle into warm bowls and swirl a spoonful of basil purée into each.

NUTRITIONAL VALUES

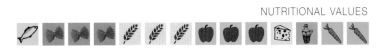

LEBANESE COUSCOUS SOUP

SERVES **6**

*Couscous, tiny grains made from semolina, is usually steamed over a stew or stock.
In this recipe, the couscous is used to thicken a richly spiced onion soup.*

4 large onions, finely sliced

3 garlic cloves, finely sliced

4 tbsp olive oil

1 red chilli, deseeded and finely chopped

1 tsp mild chilli powder

1/2 tsp ground turmeric

1 tsp ground coriander

freshly ground black pepper

2.7 litres vegetable (see page 24) or chicken stock
(see page 25)

40 g couscous

fresh coriander, chopped, to garnish

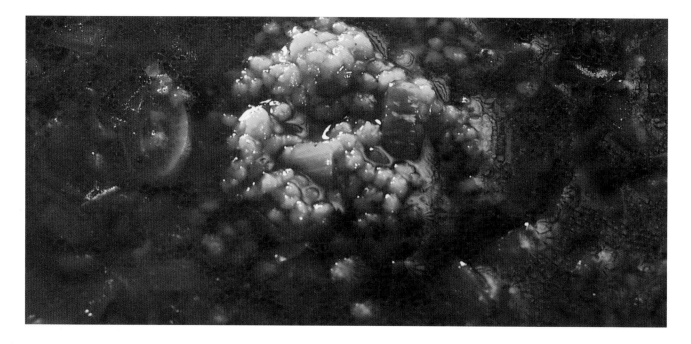

1 Cook the onions and garlic in the oil until well browned. This will take about 15 minutes over medium high heat. You must let the onions brown to achieve a rich colour for the finished soup.

2 Stir in the chopped chilli and the spices and cook over a low heat for a further 1–2 minutes before adding the stock. Season lightly then bring to the boil. Cover and simmer gently for 30 minutes.

3 Stir the couscous into the soup, return to the boil and simmer for a further 10 minutes. Season to taste, then garnish with the coriander and serve immediately.

NUTRITIONAL VALUES

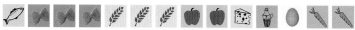

CORN CHOWDER

SERVES **4**

A lovely thick sweetcorn soup, the perfect starter for any meal.

4 slices of streaky bacon

1 medium onion, peeled and diced

1 potato, peeled and cubed

325 g can sweetcorn or frozen corn

600 ml chicken stock (see page 25)

salt substitute (see page 12) and freshly ground
  black pepper

300 ml milk

$1/4$ tsp Tabasco sauce

1 tbsp parsley, chopped

1 Remove any rind from the bacon slices and cut into small pieces.

2 On a low heat, place the bacon in a saucepan and allow to cook in its own fat. When there is a little fat in the pan, turn up the heat and allow to crisp. Add the onion and fry for 1 minute.

3 Add the potato cubes, stir round, then add half the corn with the chicken stock and seasoning. Bring to the boil and simmer for 30 minutes. Allow to cool slightly and liquidize the soup in a blender or food processor.

4 Return the saucepan and stir in the milk and the remaining corn. Heat through over a low heat. Add Tabasco sauce and taste for seasoning.

5 Sprinkle with chopped parsley.

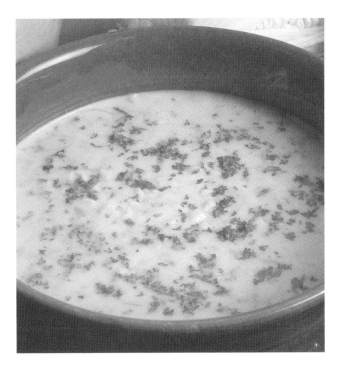

NUTRITIONAL VALUES

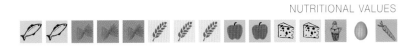

SQUASH CHOWDER

SERVES **6**

Use any hard-skinned squash for this chowder. Crown Prince is a favourite but acorn will work just as well, although a smoother-skinned squash will be easier to peel.

350 g Crown Prince squash, finely diced

2 rashers smoked back bacon, finely diced

2 tbsp fruity olive oil

4–5 sprigs fresh thyme

2 bay leaves

750 ml well-flavoured vegetable stock (see pag 24)

salt substitute (see page 12) and freshly ground

    black pepper

100 g white cabbage, finely grated

50 g creamed coconut, crumbled or diced

250 ml milk

1 large tomato, finely diced

125 g frozen prawns (optional)

1 tbsp white wine vinegar

parsley, freshly chopped, to garnish

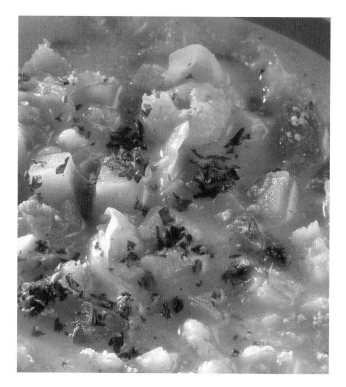

1 Cook the squash and the bacon in the oil in a heavy pan for 6–8 minutes, stirring frequently, until the squash is beginning to soften. Add the herbs and stock, season lightly, then bring to the boil. Reduce the heat and simmer for 10 minutes, then add the cabbage and creamed coconut and continue cooking for a further 10–15 minutes.

2 Remove the thyme and bay leaves, then add the milk and the chopped tomato with the prawns, if desired. Return the chowder to the boil and cook for a further 5 minutes. Season to taste then add the vinegar and parsley just before serving.

NUTRITIONAL VALUES

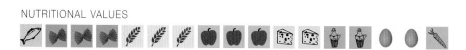

BUTTER BEAN AND MUSHROOM CHOWDER

SERVES **4**

A traditional farmhouse dish, this chowder is high in both fibre and nutrients; the butter beans are a very good source of zinc and potassium.

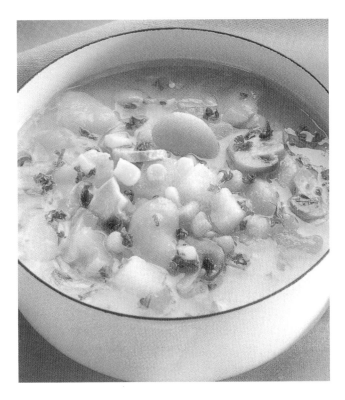

100 g butter beans, soaked overnight in cold water

1 tsp olive oil

2 medium onions, chopped

2 celery sticks, sliced

225 g potatoes, peeled or scrubbed and diced

100 g button mushrooms, trimmed and sliced

50 g tinned sweetcorn kernels, drained

300 ml skimmed milk

freshly ground black pepper

2 tbsp chopped parsley, to garnish

1 Drain the beans and place them in a large saucepan covered with fresh water. Boil them rapidly for 10 minutes, then simmer them for a further 35–40 minutes until they are soft. Drain the beans and reserve 450 ml of the stock.

2 Heat the oil in a large saucepan and fry the onion over medium heat until it softens. Add the celery and potato and cook for 2–3 minutes, stirring from time to time.

3 Add the reserved stock and mushrooms, bring to the boil then cover and simmer for 10 minutes. Add the beans, sweetcorn, and milk, bring just to simmering point and simmer for 2–3 minutes. Season to taste.

4 Serve the chowder in individual bowls, sprinkled with parsley.

NUTRITIONAL VALUES

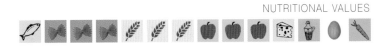

TOMATO AND ORANGE SOUP

SERVES **4**

This tangy soup is high in fibre and contains good levels of antioxidants.

700 g tomatoes, skinned and deseeded

1 potato, cubed

1 onion, sliced

1 carrot, sliced

700 ml water

1 bay leaf

juice of 1 orange

freshly ground black pepper

TO GARNISH

orange rind, finely grated

1 tbsp parsley, chopped

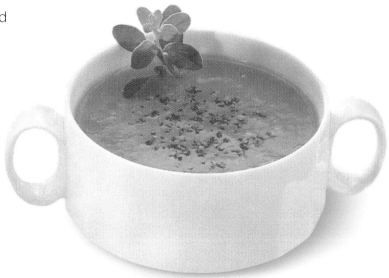

1 Place the tomatoes, potato, onion, carrot, water and bay leaf in a saucepan, bring to the boil, then simmer for about 30 minutes.

2 Remove the bay leaf and place the soup in a food processor or blender and purée until smooth.

3 Stir in the orange juice, season to taste and reheat for 1–2 minutes.

4 Mix together the orange rind and parsley, sprinkle over the soup and serve immediately.

NUTRITIONAL VALUES

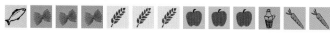

WATERCRESS SOUP

SERVES **4**

This recipe supplies vitamins and minerals, such as vitamin A, iodine, iron and calcium.

15 g unsaturated margarine

2 bunches watercress

1 onion, chopped

225 g potatoes, diced

350 g vegetable stock (see page 24)

300 ml semi-skimmed milk

pinch of cayenne pepper

salt substitute (see page 12)

TO SERVE

wholemeal toasted croûtons (optional)

NUTRITIONAL VALUES

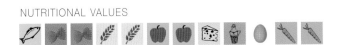

1 Melt the margarine in a large saucepan, add the onion, and cook for 2–3 minutes to soften.

2 Reserve 4 sprigs of watercress for garnish and chop the remainder. Add to the onion with the potato. Cook gently for 3–4 minutes, stirring occasionally.

3 Add the stock, bring to the boil, cover and simmer for 15–20 minutes.

4 Place in a liquidizer or food processor and blend to a purée. Return to the cleaned saucepan and add the milk and seasoning.

5 Bring to the boil and simmer for 2–3 minutes. Serve in individual soup bowls garnished with the reserved watercress sprigs.

6 If wished serve with wholemeal toasted croûtons.

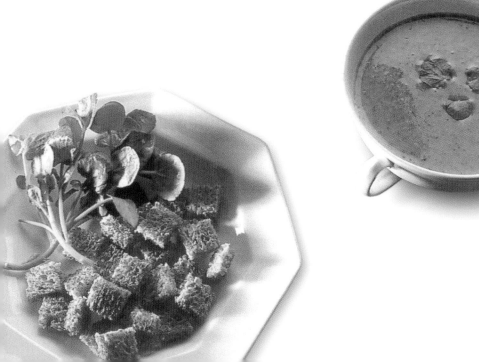

CAULIFLOWER AND SPRING ONION SOUP

SERVES **4 – 6**

A thick vegetable soup, the green onion tops providing an appealing garnish. No herbs, spices or stock are required – the flavour of the cauliflower and the onions is more than enough.

1 bunch spring onions (about 8–10), trimmed

2 tbsp butter

1 large potato, peeled and diced

1 large cauliflower, chopped (including the stalk)

1.2 litres water

salt substitute (see page 12) and freshly ground black
   pepper

250 ml milk, or more

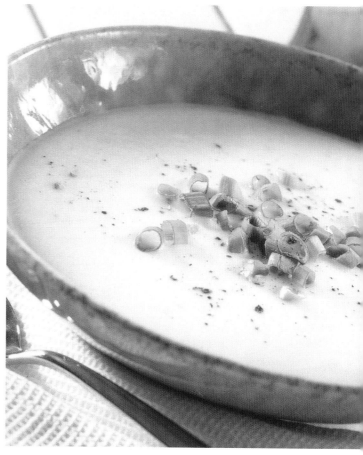

1   Reserve the green tops of the spring onions. Chop the white part and add to the butter in a pot and cook slowly for 5 minutes, until the onions are softened.

2   Stir in the potato and cauliflower, cover and cook over low heat for a further 5 minutes, shaking the pot from time to time.

3   Add the water with the pepper and bring to the boil. Cover the pot, then simmer for 20 minutes.

4   Remove from the heat and allow the soup to cool slightly then purée until smooth. Return to the stove and add the milk, thinning the soup to the required consistency. Reheat gently, seasoning to taste.

5   Finely chop the reserved green onion tops and stir into the soup just before serving.

NUTRITIONAL VALUES

PASTA GREEN SOUP

SERVES **4 – 6**

A nutritious meal in itself – low-fat and full of protein. Serve with warm, crusty garlic bread.

2 tbsp olive oil

3 cloves garlic, crushed

4 tbsp fresh parsley, chopped

150 g dried wholemeal gnocchi piccoli (shells)

1.5 litres vegetable stock (see page 24)

3 tbsp vegetable or tomato purée

400 g can mixed beans, such as borlotti, kidney, cannellini etc, drained

salt substitute (see page 12) and freshly ground black pepper

Parmesan cheese, freshly grated, to serve

1 Heat the oil in a large saucepan and sauté the garlic with the chopped parsley for about 2 minutes. Add the gnocchi piccoli and cook for 1–2 minutes, stirring constantly.

2 Pour in the vegetable stock and add the vegetable or tomato paste. Bring to the boil, reduce the heat then simmer for about 10 minutes, stirring occasionally, until the pasta is tender.

3 Add the beans and season with salt substitute and freshly ground black pepper. Continue to cook for a further 5 minutes, then serve with a little freshly grated Parmesan cheese.

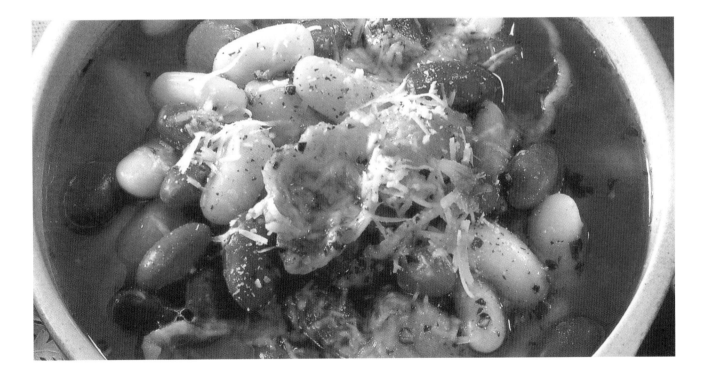

NUTRITIONAL VALUES

MEXICAN BEAN SOUP

SERVES **6**

Pinto beans are the traditional beans for Mexican cookery, but they have been replaced in many dishes by red kidney beans, which are a more attractive colour. If you are unable to get the pintos, use just kidney beans to make this thick and spicy soup.

100 g red kidney beans, soaked overnight

100 g pinto beans, soaked overnight

1 large onion, finely chopped

1 tbsp oil

1 red chilli, deseeded and finely chopped

1 large clove garlic, finely sliced

1 tsp mild chilli powder

1 tbsp coriander leaves

1.5 litre well-flavoured vegetable stock
(see page 24)

1 tbsp tomato purée

freshly ground black pepper

40 g Cheddar cheese, grated

guacamole for serving

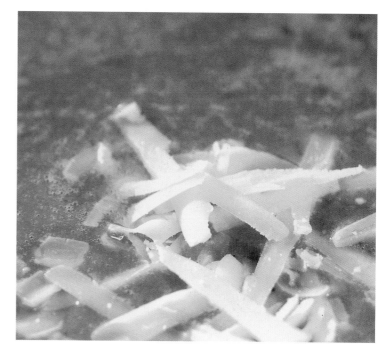

1 Drain the beans and rinse them thoroughly under cold running water, then set aside until needed. Cook the onion in the oil until soft, then add the chilli, garlic and chilli powder and cook for another minute.

2 Stir the beans into the pan then add the coriander, stock, tomato purée and seasonings. Bring the soup to the boil and boil for 10 minutes, then simmer slowly for 45–60 minutes, until the beans are soft. Allow the soup to cool, then purée until smooth in a blender or food processor. Rinse the pan then return the soup to it and reheat gently, seasoning to taste with pepper.

3 Scatter the cheese over the soup just before serving and set out a dish of guacamole.

NUTRITIONAL VALUES

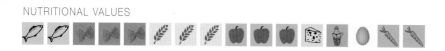

DEVILS ON HORSEBACK

makeS **12**

These are simple to prepare and can be made earlier and kept in the fridge if you don't have much time.

12 prunes, soaked
6 slices streaky bacon
12 tooth picks

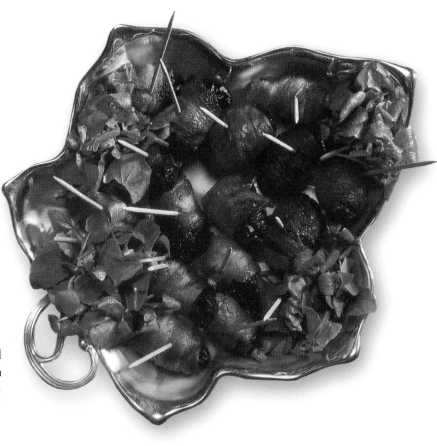

1 Place the soaked prunes in a small saucepan covered with water, bring to the boil and simmer for 5 minutes. Drain and allow to cool slightly.

2 Remove the stones from the prunes and reshape.

3 Cut the rind from the bacon, cut each slice in half and smooth out with a spatula. Place a piece of foil on the grill and arrange the slices of bacon on the foil. Cook for 2 minutes under a hot grill. Do not allow to crisp.

4 When slightly cooled, wrap the bacon pieces around the prunes and finish cooking under the grill or in the oven if more convenient.

5 Secure with tooth picks. Serve as an appetizer with pre-dinner drinks.

NUTRITIONAL VALUES

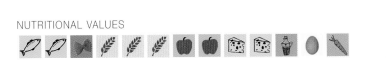

ROASTED TOMATO TARTLETS

SERVES **6**

Serve these tartlets hot or cold with a crisp green salad on the side.

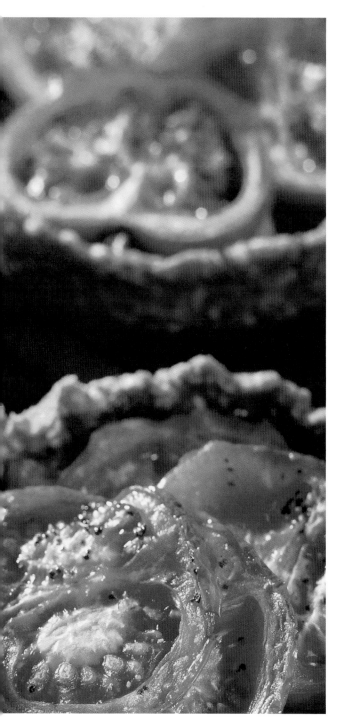

DOUGH

250 g fine wholemeal flour

25 g sesame seeds

1/2 tsp salt substitute (see page 12)

1 large egg, beaten

5 tbsp olive oil

3–4 tbsp water

TOMATO FILLING

3 onions, finely sliced

2 cloves garlic , halved

3 tbsp fruit olive oil

3–4 sprigs fresh thyme

2 bay leaves

freshly ground black pepper

4–5 large tomatoes, sliced

1 Mix together flour, sesame seeds and salt substitute, then make a well in the centre. Add egg and olive oil and mix to a soft dough, adding water as necessary. Divide mixture into six and shape to line six 10 cm individual tart dishes – this is more of a dough than a pastry and is easiest to mold into shape with your fingers. Chill tart shells for at least 30 minutes while preparing tartlet filling.

2 Cook onions and garlic in olive oil with thyme and bay leaves for 30–40 minutes, until well softened and reduced. Season to taste, then remove herbs from pan.

3 Preheat oven to 220°C/gas mark 7. Fill tart shells with onion mixture then top with tomatoes, overlapping the slices and brushing them lightly with olive oil. Season well with pepper, then bake in a preheated oven for 20–25 minutes, until dough is crisp and tomatoes are just starting to blacken. Serve hot or cold with a crisp, green leaf salad on the side.

NUTRITIONAL VALUES

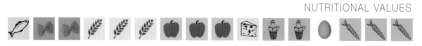

BRAISED CHESTNUTS WITH ONIONS AND PRUNES

SERVES **6**

A vegetarian starter that can be prepared the day before if you don't have much time.

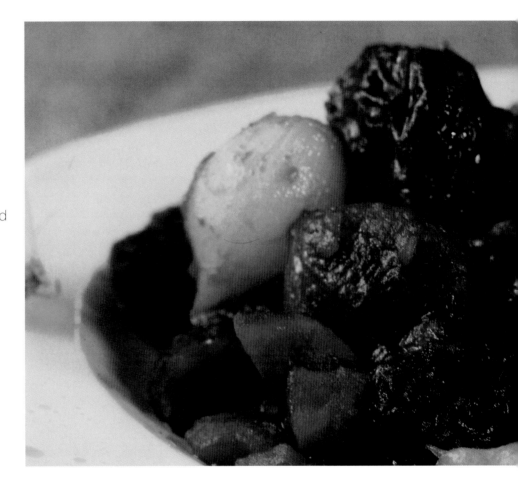

1 tbsp olive oil

450 g chestnuts, shelled and
peeled

450 g small white onions, peeled

500 ml beef stock

250 ml good-quality port wine

45 g firmly packed soft dark
brown sugar

1 bay leaf

225 g pitted prunes

freshly ground black pepper to
taste

1   In a large, heavy sauté pan, heat the oil and sauté the chestnuts until lightly browned, about 7 minutes. Remove with a slotted spoon and reserve.

2   Sauté the onions until lightly browned, about 5–7 minutes. Return the chestnuts to the pan and add the stock, port, brown sugar, and bay leaf. Bring to the boil, then lower the heat and simmer for 30 minutes, stirring gently several times. Add the prunes and return to a simmer. Continue to simmer, stirring gently several times, for 30–35 minutes more or until the liquid has formed a syrupy glaze.

3   Remove the bay leaf, season to taste with pepper and serve hot. This recipe may be made a day in advance and reheated by adding 125 ml more stock and cooking on low heat until the syrupy glaze has re-formed.

NUTRITIONAL VALUES

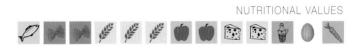

SPINACH TOMATOES

SERVES **4**

These spinach stuffed tomatoes are served garnished with breadcrumbs and cheese and a few green leaves.

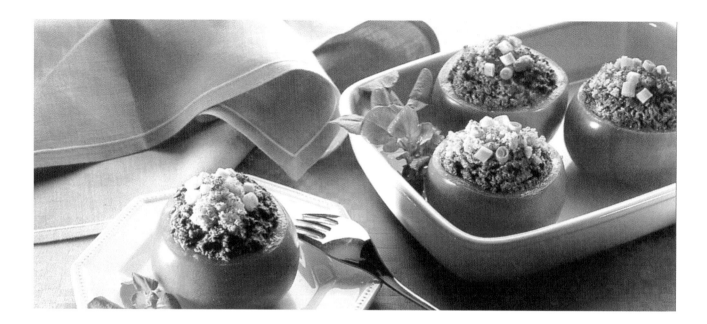

4 large tomatoes

225 g fresh spinach

2 tbsp strained Greek yoghurt

$\frac{1}{2}$ tsp nutmeg, freshly grated

salt substitute (see page 12) and freshly ground
   black pepper

2 spring onions, sliced into rings

1 tbsp toasted wholemeal breadcrumbs

1 tbsp Parmesan cheese, grated

1 Slice the tops off the tomatoes and scoop out the insides, taking care not to cut through the tomato shell.

2 Wash the spinach and place, wet, in a saucepan. Cook for 2–3 minutes over a medium heat until it softens, stirring continuously.

3 Drain the spinach, squeeze out any excess moisture and chop finely. Mix with the yoghurt, nutmeg and seasoning.

4 Reserve a few spring onion rings and add the remainder to the spinach and mix together.

5 Spoon the mix into the tomatoes. Mix together the breadcrumbs and cheese and sprinkle over the top.

NUTRITIONAL VALUES

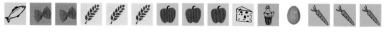

STUFFED PASTA SHELLS

SERVES **4 – 6**

These are great as a starter or served as a canapé with drinks at a party. They can be made in advance and served cold or reheated in the oven to serve warm.

12 dried conchiglie rigate (large shells)

dash of olive oil

FOR THE FILLING

225 g brown lentils, washed and drained

2 cloves of garlic, crushed

400 g can chopped tomatoes

1 tbsp tomato purée

3 tbsp fresh basil, chopped

50 ml dry red wine

freshly ground black pepper

FOR THE TOPPING

25 g fine dried breadcrumbs

25 g Parmesan cheese, finely grated

3 tbsp fresh parsley, chopped

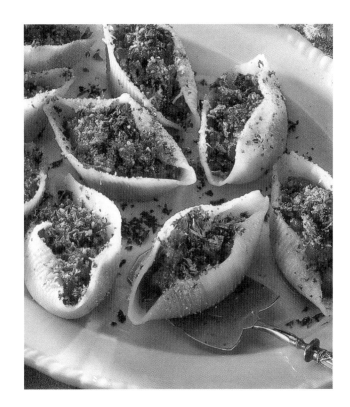

1 Bring a large saucepan of water to the boil and add the conchiglie rigate with a dash of olive oil. Cook for about 10 minutes, stirring occasionally, until tender. Drain and rinse under cold running water. Drain again and lay out on absorbent kitchen paper.

2 To make the filling, bring a large saucepan of water to the boil and add the lentils. Simmer for about 30 minutes, until tender. Drain and rinse under boiling water.

3 Place the garlic, chopped tomatoes, tomato purée, fresh basil, wine and freshly ground black pepper in a large frying pan. Bring to boiling point, then reduce the heat and simmer for 2–3 minutes. Add the lentils, stir and cook for about 10 minutes, until the moisture has evaporated and the mixture has thickened.

4 Use a teaspoon to stuff the pasta shells with the filling mixture and arrange them on a baking sheet. Combine the topping ingredients in a small bowl and sprinkle over the stuffed shells. Place under a hot grill for about 5 minutes, until golden.

NUTRITIONAL VALUES

CORN ON THE COB WITH GARLIC BUTTER

A delicious way to serve sweetcorn, make sure you have a napkin handy as this is finger-licking good!

4 pieces of fresh corn

garlic butter

olive oil

salt substitute (see page 12) and freshly ground
  black pepper

1 Remove the outer green leaves from the fresh corn. Place in boiling salted water with a drop of olive oil.

2 Simmer for 20 minutes, or until the corn is cooked and tender.

3 Remove from the heat and drain.

4 Smother liberally with garlic butter.

5 Sprinkle with salt substitute and freshly ground black pepper.

NUTRITIONAL VALUES

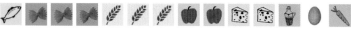

MAIN COURSES

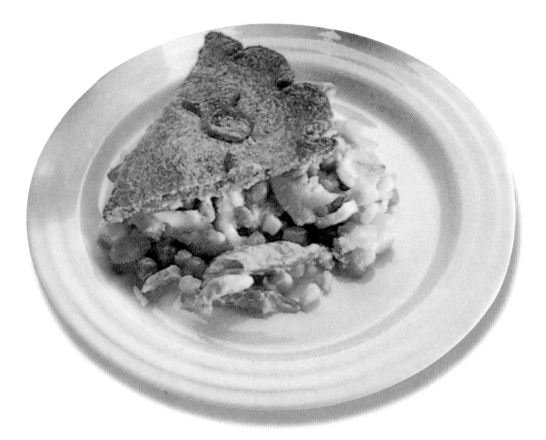

LENTIL AND CORIANDER LASAGNE

SERVES **1**

You could make up two or three portions and freeze them uncooked. They cook beautifully from frozen at 190˚C/gas mark 5 for 50–60 minutes.

75 g red lentils, washed and drained

1 onion, roughly chopped

425 ml boiling water

1 tbsp olive oil, plus extra for greasing

1 clove garlic, crushed

3 tbsp fresh coriander, chopped

75 g mushrooms, sliced

2 tsp sweet soya sauce

1 tbsp tomato purée

salt substitute (see page 12) and freshly ground
   black pepper

1 sheet fresh lasagne (approx 20 x 10 cm) cut
   in half

¹/₂ quantity of cheese sauce

75 g red Leicester cheese, grated

1 Place the lentils and chopped onion in a large saucepan and add the boiling water. Bring to the boil, then simmer for about 15 minutes. Drain and set aside. Preheat the oven to 200˚C/gas mark 6.

2 Heat the olive oil in a large frying pan and sauté the garlic and coriander for about a minute, then add the sliced mushrooms. Cook for about 4 minutes then add the sweet soya sauce and tomato purée and season with salt substitute and freshly ground black pepper. Add the cooked lentil mixture, stir, and cook gently for about 5 minutes.

3 To assemble the lasagne, oil a shallow ovenproof dish and place one sheet of the lasagne on the bottom. Cover with half the lentil mixture, then add the other sheet of lasagne. Spoon the remaining lentil mixture over the top, spread out evenly, then pour the cheese sauce over the top. Sprinkle with grated cheese then bake for about 20 minutes.

NUTRITIONAL VALUES

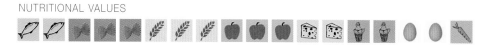

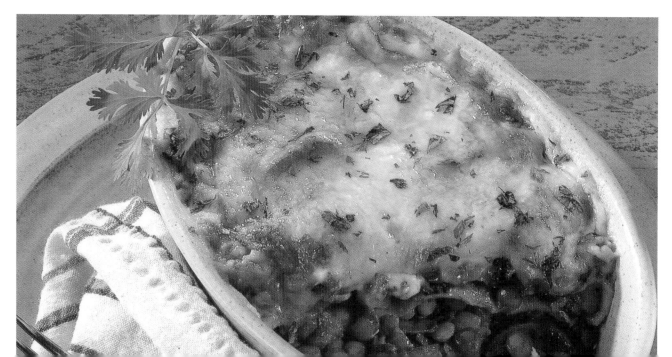

CRACKED WHEAT PILAU

SERVES **4**

A very coarse cracked wheat is often used in this dish as it gives a good, nutty texture. The wheat makes a welcome change from rice.

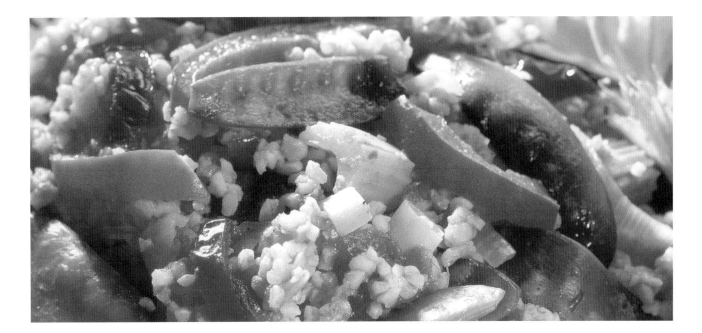

1 large onion, sliced

1 leek, trimmed and sliced

2 tbsp olive oil

1 tsp ground cumin

1 tsp ground ginger

1–2 plump cloves garlic, finely sliced

4 sticks celery, trimmed and sliced

1 red pepper, deseeded and sliced

125 g baby corn, halved

225 g cracked wheat

400 g tin chopped tomatoes

700 ml water or vegetable stock (see page 24)

salt substitute (see page 12) and freshly ground
   black pepper

125 g mange tout, topped and tailed

6 halves sun-dried tomatoes, grated

1   Cook the onion and leek in the oil until softened but not browned, then add the spices and cook for another minute. Add the garlic, celery, pepper and corn, then cook briefly before stirring the cracked wheat into the pan. Add the tomatoes, stock and seasonings, then simmer for 12–15 minutes, stirring occasionally. Add the mange tout and sun-dried tomatoes and cook for a further 4–5 minutes. Serve with a tossed green salad.

NUTRITIONAL VALUES

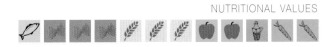

PASTA WITH SPINACH SAUCE

SERVES **4**

This creamy pasta dish is great for entertaining, serve topped with Parmesan cheese and accompanied with a crisp green salad.

300 g wholemeal or spinach pasta shapes

1 kg fresh spinach

2 tbsp olive oil

1 onion, chopped

2 cloves garlic, chopped

175 g mushrooms, sliced

250 g ricotta or cream cheese

1–2 tbsp pine kernels

freshly ground black pepper

Parmesan cheese, grated

1 Wash spinach and discard tough stalks. Pack into a large pan, cover, and cook over a low heat until soft, stirring occasionally. Drain and chop.

2 Heat oil in a pan and fry the onions and garlic until soft. Stir in the mushrooms. Cover and cook over a low heat until soft.

3 Mix the vegetables with the cheese and pine kernels and season to taste. Keep warm.

4 Cook the pasta in plenty of boiling water until soft but firm to the bite. Drain. Stir sauce into pasta and serve. Offer Parmesan cheese.

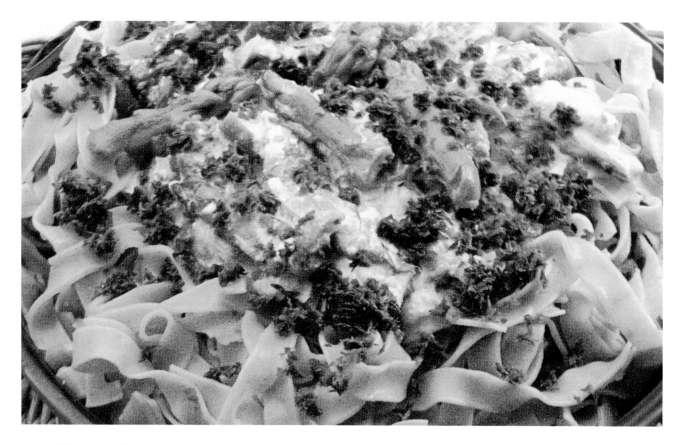

NUTRITIONAL VALUES

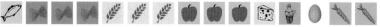

MIXED MASALA BEANS

SERVES **4**

Not only do the ingredients blend very well together, they also make a very | colourful dish.

1 tbsp olive oil

50 g onion, chopped

1/2 tsp cumin seeds

1/2 tsp chilli powder

1/4 tsp turmeric

1/4 tsp garam masala

225 g chickpeas, canned, drained

225 g kidney beans, canned, drained

50 g tomatoes, chopped

1–2 green chillies, chopped

4 cloves garlic

1 tsp grated ginger

100 g green peppers, chopped

2 tsp lemon juice

2–3 tbsp coriander leaves, chopped

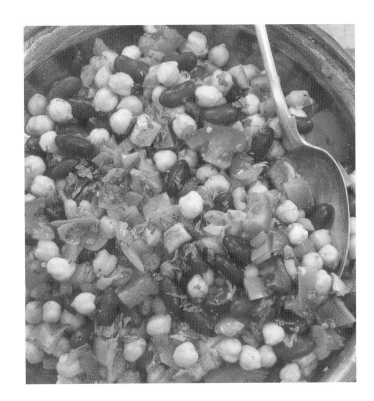

1 Heat the oil in a medium-size heavy saucepan, then stir in the onion and cumin seeds and fry them until the onions turn a light gold colour.

2 Add the chilli powder, turmeric and garam masala and stir. Add 2 tablespoons of water and cook, stirring continuously for a minute or so.

3 Gently stir in the chickpeas, kidney beans, tomato, green chillies, garlic, and ginger. Mix well and stir in 240 ml of water. Bring to the boil, then reduce the heat and simmer for 15–20 minutes.

4 Add the green pepper and cook for 2–3 minutes more.

5 Stir in the lemon juice and half the coriander leaves. Use the remaining coriander leaves to garnish the dish.

NUTRITIONAL VALUES

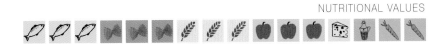

DEEP-DISH CREOLE PIZZA

MAKES 33 x 22 cm deep pan pizza

Creole dishes tend to be spicy tomato and vegetable mixtures, and this pizza is no exception. You can try using fresh okra if it is available. Boil the whole fresh okra until tender. Then chop it to use in this recipe.

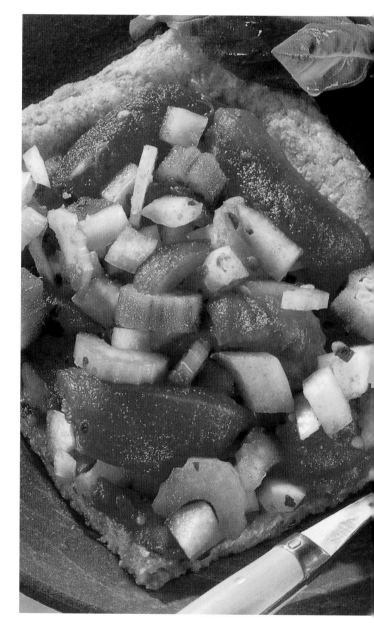

½ quantity wholemeal pizza dough (see
   page 55)

2 x 400 g can tomatoes

1 tsp oregano

1 tsp thyme

½ tsp basil

½ tsp cayenne pepper

2 cloves garlic, crushed

2 celery stalks, chopped

1 small onion, chopped

225 g cut frozen okra, thawed

1   Preheat the oven to 250°C/gas mark 10.

2   Place the dough in the centre of a lightly oiled 33 x 22 x 5 cm pan. Using your fingers, spread the dough until it covers the bottom of the pan evenly and goes halfway up the sides.

3   Put the tomatoes into a colander, drain, and discard the liquid but retain the thick sauce. Cut the tomatoes into quarters. Place the tomatoes and sauce in a bowl. Add the herbs, spice, and garlic. Chop the celery and onions into small pieces and add them to the bowl. Finally, add the okra and stir gently to mix.

4   To assemble, spread the tomato and okra mixture onto the pizza dough and bake for 20 minutes.

NUTRITIONAL VALUES

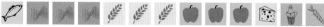

FETTUCINE PRIMAVERA

SERVES **4**

Fresh baby vegetables have a flavour all their own. In this dish they are served simply, with a yoghurt and garlic sauce and plain pasta. Use any combination of mixed vegetables that you have to hand for a spur-of-the-moment dish.

300 g fettucine

75 g broccoli florets

4 baby carrots, halved lengthways

1 medium red pepper, cubed

1 medium green pepper, cubed

1 medium red onion, quartered and thinly sliced

50 g broad beans

25 g peas

2 cloves garlic, peeled and crushed

6 tbsp freshly grated Cheddar cheese

5 tbsp plain yoghurt

pinch of cayenne pepper

salt substitute (see page 12)

1 Bring a large quantity of water to the boil in the base of the steamer and add the pasta.

2 Place all of the vegetables in a waxed paper-lined steamer tier, cover with a tight-fitting lid, and steam over the pasta for 10 minutes. Check the pasta before 10 minutes to ensure it does not overcook.

3 Add the cheese, yoghurt, and cayenne pepper to the vegetables and keep warm.

4 Drain the pasta and transfer to a warm serving dish. Top with the vegetables, season well, and serve immediately.

NUTRITIONAL VALUES

PASTA WITH GREEN PEPPERS AND PESTO

SERVES **4**

If linguini is unavailable, spaghettini or tagliatelle will work just as well in this dish.

450 g fresh linguini (thin, flat strips)

dash of olive oil, plus 2 tbsp

2 cloves garlic, crushed

$^{1}/_{2}$ quantity pesto sauce

50 ml vegetable stock (see page 24)

1 green pepper, deseeded and very thinly sliced

fresh herbs, to garnish

1 Bring a large saucepan of water to the boil and add the linguini with a dash of olive oil. Cook for about 4 minutes, stirring occasionally, until tender. Drain and return to the saucepan. Stir in a dash more olive oil and set aside, covered, to keep warm.

2 Heat the remaining olive oil in a large frying pan and sauté the garlic for 1–2 minutes, then stir in the pesto sauce. Add the vegetable stock, stir, and cook for 1 minute, then add the pepper slices. Cook for a further 7–10 minutes, stirring occasionally, until the pepper has softened. Stir the pepper mixture into the linguini and serve, garnished with fresh herbs.

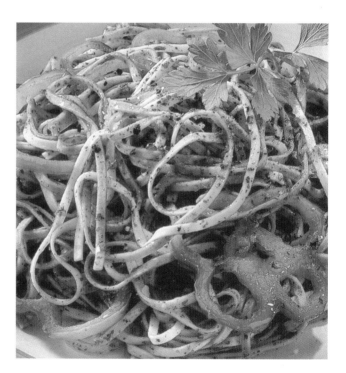

NUTRITIONAL VALUES

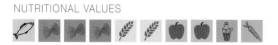

PEPPER AND PASTA RATATOUILLE

SERVES **4 – 6**

Delicious served with a hot, buttered baked potato, this dish makes perfect bonfire-night fare.

450 g dried wholemeal gnocchi piccoli (small
    shells)

dash of olive oil, plus 3 tbsp

2 cloves garlic, minced

1 onion, chopped

2 green peppers, deseeded and cut into chunks

400 g can chopped tomatoes

50 g tomato purée

150 ml dry red wine

2 tbsp fresh oregano

salt and freshly ground black pepper

fresh oregano sprigs, to garnish

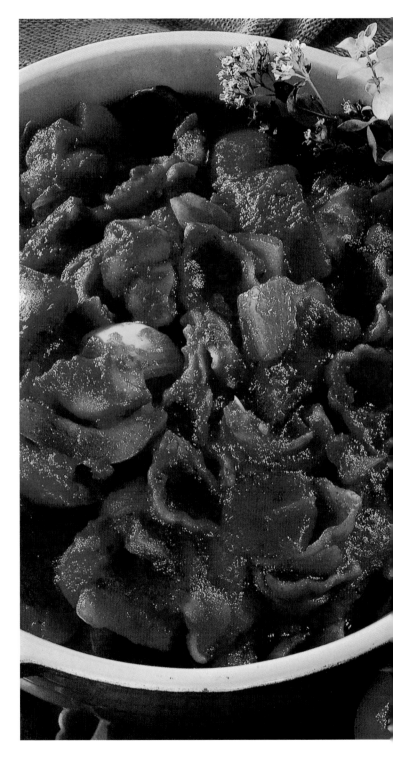

1   Bring a large saucepan of water to the boil and add the gnocchi piccoli with a dash of olive oil. Cook for about 10 minutes, stirring occasionally, until tender. Drain and set aside.

2   Heat the remaining olive oil in a large saucepan and sauté the garlic and onion for about 3 minutes, until softened. Stir in the pepper chunks. Cover and cook for about 5 minutes, or until the pepper has softened slightly.

3   Stir in the remaining ingredients, except the oregano sprigs, into the pepper mixture and bring to simmering point. Reduce the heat, cover and cook for about 10 minutes, then stir in the gnocchi piccoli. Cook for a further 5 minutes, stirring occasionally. Serve garnished with fresh oregano sprigs.

NUTRITIONAL VALUES

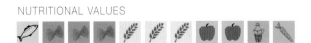

FUSILLI WITH ROASTED PEPPERS

SERVES **4 – 6**

To prevent the pasta from sticking together, wash off the starchy cooking liquid by rinsing the pasta under boiling water from the kettle. Continue as directed in the recipe.

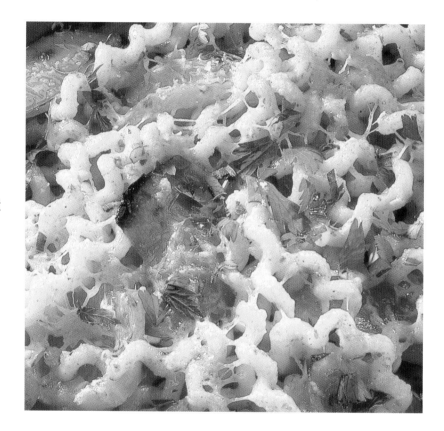

450 g dried long fusilli

dash of olive oil

2 yellow peppers, deseeded and cut into chunks

3 cloves of garlic, minced

50 ml olive oil

100 g grated Cheddar cheese

100 g freshly grated Parmesan cheese

chopped fresh parsley, to garnish

1 Bring a large saucepan of water to the boil and add the fusilli with a dash of olive oil. Cook for about 10 minutes, stirring occasionally, until tender. Drain, return to the saucepan and set aside.

2 Preheat the oven to 200°C/gas mark 6. Arrange the chunks of pepper on a baking sheet and place under a hot grill for about 5 minutes, or until slightly charred.

3 Mix the pepper into the pasta with the remaining ingredients and toss together to combine. Transfer to an ovenproof dish and bake for about 15 minutes, or until heated through and the cheese has melted. Sprinkle over the chopped parsley and serve.

NUTRITIONAL VALUES

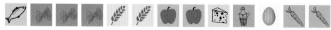

CABBAGE WITH PASTA MOLD

SERVES **4 – 6**

Serve as an impressive dish for family or friends. Quick and easy to prepare, your guests will certainly be impressed.

175 g dried wholemeal macaroni

dash of olive oil, plus extra for greasing

175 g small cauliflour florets

275 ml Tomato Sauce

15 g grated Parmesan cheese

50 g grated mature Cheddar cheese

2 tbsp chopped fresh parsley

freshly ground black pepper

5 large savoy cabbage leaves, stalks removed

fresh herbs, to garnish

1 Bring a large saucepan of water to the boil and add the macaroni with a dash of olive oil. Cook for about 10 minutes, stirring occasionally, until tender. Drain and set aside.

2 Meanwhile, blanch the cauliflour florets in boiling water, drain, and place in a bowl. Stir in the macaroni, tomato Sauce, Parmesan and Cheddar cheeses, chopped parsley, and season with freshly ground black pepper. Allow to cool completely.

3 Preheat the oven to 180°C/gas mark 4. Blanch the cabbage leaves in boiling water, then drain and rinse under cold running water immediately. Pat dry with absorbent kitchen paper, then use to line a 1 l greased pudding basin, overlapping the leaves and covering the base. Allow the leaves to hang over the sides of the basin.

4 Spoon the cool pasta mixture into the prepared basin, pressing down firmly with the back of the spoon. Fold the overhanging leaves over the top to encase the pasta filling. Cover the top of the basin with greased aluminium foil and bake in the centre of the oven for about 25–30 minutes. Leave to stand for 10 minutes before inverting on to a serving plate. Garnish with fresh herbs and serve.

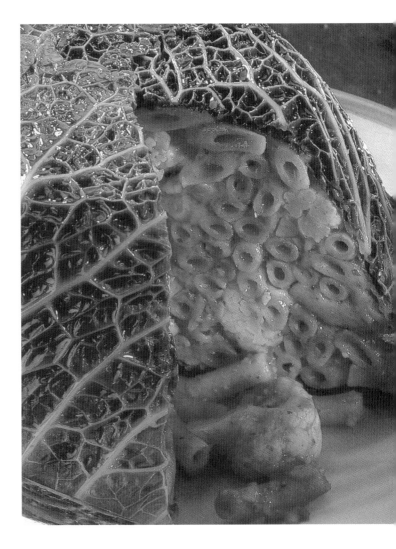

NUTRITIONAL VALUES

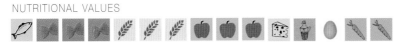

BLUE CHEESE AND BROCCOLI PIZZA

MAKES **30-cm double crust pizza**

When creamy blue cheese melts on the top of this pizza, it turns ordinary broccoli into a treat. The pecans add to the delight.

¹/₂ quantity garlic dill pizza dough

FOR THE TOPPING

1 small head of broccoli,
    separated into florets

1 small white onion, thinly sliced

1 tbsp olive oil

50 g pecans, chopped

100 g blue cheese, crumbled

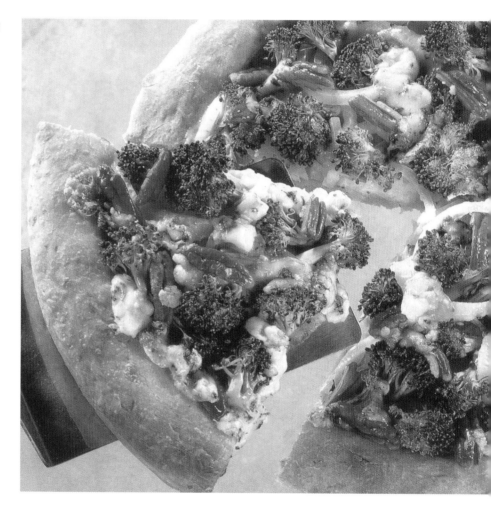

1   Preheat oven to 250°C/gas mark 10.

2   Remove the stem from the broccoli; separate the head into small florets. You need about 225 g. To assemble the pizza, first lay the thinly sliced onion over the pizza dough. Then add the broccoli. Sprinkle the olive oil over the vegetables. Add the pecans and top with the crumbled blue cheese.

3   Bake in the lower half of the oven for about 6 minutes.

NUTRITIONAL VALUES

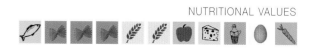

LENTIL MOUSSAKA

SERVES **4–6**

A meatless variation of the classic baked dish. This is rich, filling and full of fibre, so it must be good for you!

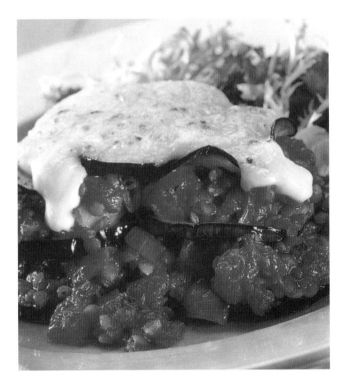

olive oil, for frying

1 large onion, chopped

2 cloves garlic, chopped

2 cloves garlic, crushed

1 green pepper, cored and chopped

150 g red lentils

about 170 ml red wine

300 g canned chopped tomatoes

salt substitute (see page 12) and freshly ground
   black pepper

1 tbsp chopped fresh oregano

2 large aubergines, sliced

625 ml milk

4 tbsp butter, plus extra for greasing

4 tbsp all-purpose flour

1 cup Cheddar cheese, grated

1 Preheat a 220°C/Gas mark 7 oven. In a large pan heat 2 tablespoons of oil. Add the onion, garlic and pepper and cook gently until soft. Add the lentils, red wine, and tomatoes. Bring to the boil, then season and add the oregano. Simmer for 20 minutes, or until the lentils are soft. Add a little more wine to the sauce if it seems dry.

2 Meanwhile, heat 2–3 tablespoons of oil in a frying pan. Fry the aubergine slices on both sides until tender, adding more oil if necessary, then drain on paper towels. Add any oil left in the frying pan to the lentil sauce.

3 Heat the milk, butter, and flour in a pan, stirring all the time, until boiling and thickened. Continue to cook for 1 minute, to remove the taste of flour from the sauce, then remove the pan from the heat. Add all but 2 tablespoons of the grated cheese and then season to taste.

4 Layer the lentil sauce and aubergine slices in a buttered, ovenproof dish, finishing with a layer of aubergine. Spoon the sauce over the aubergine, then scatter the remaining cheese over the top. Bake in the preheated for 30 minutes, until the moussaka is browned and set. Serve with a salad and garlic bread.

NUTRITIONAL VALUES

ROASTED RED PEPPER PITA BREAD

Roasted red pepper, kneaded into the dough, gives this flatbread an unusual flavour. Homemade pita bread tastes good made on the barbecue.

2 tsp dried yeast

pinch sugar

150 ml warm water, or as needed

450 g unbleached white flour

1 tbsp fresh thyme

1 tsp salt substitute (see page 12)

1 tbsp extra-virgin olive oil, plus a little extra

2 red peppers, roasted, peeled and chopped

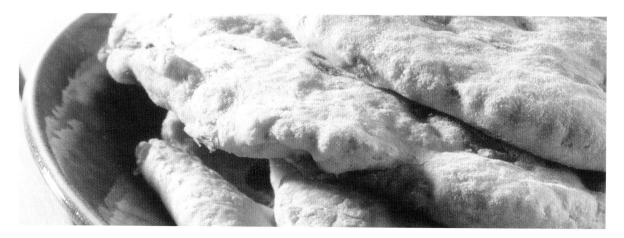

1 Dissolve the yeast with the sugar in about 125 ml of warm water and leave for about 10 minutes or until frothy. If it fails to froth, start again (your yeast may be old or the temperature of the room may be too cool).

2 In a large bowl, mix the flour with the thyme, salt substitute and oil, then add the yeast, remaining water and red peppers and begin mixing with a fork. When it gets too hard to mix with a fork, start kneading with your hands on a floured board. Knead for about 10 minutes or until smooth and elastic.

3 Pour the olive oil into a large bowl and swirl it around to coat the sides. Place the dough in this bowl, cover with plastic wrap and leave in a warm place for about an hour and a half, or until doubled in size.

4 Punch the dough down, and divide it into 6 equal pieces. Roll out each piece on a lightly floured board with a floured rolling pin until about 20 cm in diameter and about 5 mm thick.

5 Arrange them on a floured surface such as a board or plates and leave for about 30 minutes or until they have risen slightly and are puffy.

6 Preheat the oven to 220°C/gas mark 7.

7 Transfer the pitas to ungreased non-stick baking sheets and bake for 8–10 minutes or until puffed up and lightly golden. It is better to underbake rather than overbake pitas.

NUTRITIONAL VALUES

FISH AND SWEETCORN PIE

SERVES **4**

There is a pleasing affinity of flavours between fresh or smoked fish and sweetcorn, the principal ingredients in this tasty pie filling.

PASTRY

175 g wholemeal flour

1 tsp mustard powder

75 g unsaturated margarine

FILLING

1 tbsp olive oil

1 medium onion, chopped

15 g wholemeal flour

150 ml skimmed milk

2 tbsp parsley, chopped

$1/4$ tsp ground mace

freshly ground black pepper

225 g smoked haddock, cooked, skinned and flaked

100 g frozen peas, thawed

100 g canned sweetcorn kernels, drained

GLAZE

beaten egg or milk

1 Set the oven to 200°C/gas mark 6. To make the pastry, place the flour and mustard in a large bowl, add the margarine and rub together until the mixture resembles fine breadcrumbs. Add just enough cold water to mix to a smooth dough. Wrap and chill for 20 minutes.

2 To make the filling, pour the oil into a saucepan and cook the onion over medium heat for about 3 minutes to soften it. Stir in the flour and cook, stirring, for a few seconds. Gradually add the milk, continuing to stir all the time, bring the sauce to the boil. Add the parsley, mace, seasoning, fish, peas and sweetcorn, and heat through. Transfer the mixture to a pie dish.

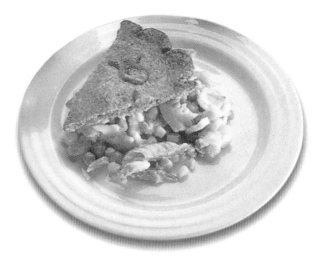

3 Roll out the pastry to fit the dish. Cover the filling with the pastry and make a slit in the centre to allow the steam to escape. Pinch the edges to make a decorative pattern and use the pastry trimmings to decorate the pie top. Brush the pastry with beaten egg or milk.

4 Bake the pie in the oven for 30 minutes, or until the pastry is golden. A green salad is a good accompaniment.

NUTRITIONAL VALUES

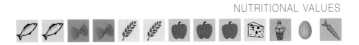

SPICED BEAN CHICKEN

SERVES **4**

This Eastern feast is full of protein and fibre. It can be served with some naan bread and a crisp fresh salad.

175 g mixed dried pulses (red kidney beans, chickpeas, haricot beans, etc.)

1 clove garlic, finely chopped

1 medium onion, finely chopped

2 tbsp olive oil

$\frac{1}{2}$ tsp turmeric

$\frac{1}{2}$ tsp ground cumin

8 medium chicken drumsticks

freshly ground black pepper

6 tomatoes, deseeded and chopped

600 ml chicken stock (see page 25)

100 g okra (ladies fingers)

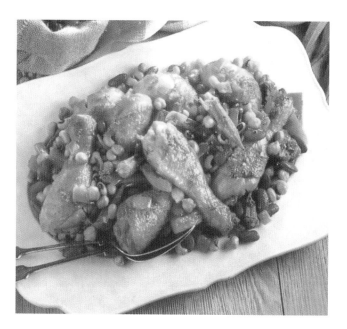

1 Soak the pulses in cold water overnight. Drain and put into a pan with enough fresh cold water to cover well, and boil steadily for 10 minutes. Drain thoroughly.

2 Heat the oil in a large saucepan, add the onion and garlic and cook gently until softened.

3 Add the spices and cook for a further minute than add the chicken drumsticks. Season to taste. Cook, stirring for 5 minutes until the chicken is coated with the spices.

4 Add the tomatoes, stock, and drained pulses, cover and simmer gently for 45–60 minutes or until the beans are tender.

5 Add the okra (ladies fingers) 5 minutes before the end of cooking.

6 Serve piping hot sprinkled with fresh chopped parsley.

NUTRITIONAL VALUES

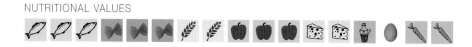

BUCKWHEAT STUFFED ROAST CHICKEN

SERVES **4 – 6**

This tasty dish is served with a little of the gravy poured over the chicken.

175 g roasted buckwheat

475 ml water

1 onion, finely chopped

1 tbsp olive oil

1 clove garlic, crushed (optional)

100 g chicken livers, chopped

1/2 tsp dried marjoram (oregano)

freshly ground black pepper

1 egg, beaten

1.5 kg oven-ready chicken

DILL STUFFING

1 small onion, finely chopped

1 tbsp olive oil

175 g fresh white breadcrumbs

4 tbsp fresh dill, chopped

2 eggs

salt substitute (see page 12) and
    freshly ground black pepper

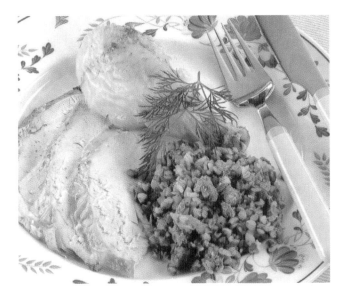

1 Place the buckwheat in a sieve and rinse under cold running water. Put the buckwheat in a saucepan and pour in the water. Heat very gently until the water is just about simmering. Remove the pan from the heat, cover and leave for 30 minutes by which time the buckwheat should have absorbed all the water.

2 Cook the onion in the oil for 10 minutes, until soft but not browned. Add the garlic and chicken livers and cook for a further 5 minutes, stirring occasionally, until the pieces of liver are firm. Add this mixture to the buckwheat with the marjoram and seasoning to taste. Stir in the egg to bind, making sure all the ingredients are thoroughly combined.

3 To make a dill stuffing, cook the small, chopped onion in the oil until soft. Mix the onion with the breadcrumbs, the chopped fresh dill, freshly ground black pepper and 2 egg yolks. Whisk the whites until they peak softly, then stir into the stuffing.

4 Set the oven at 180°C/gas mark 4. Rinse the chicken under cold running water, drain well and pat dry with absorbent kitchen paper towel. Spoon the stuffing into the body cavity and truss the bird neatly, tying string around the legs and wings. Place in a roasting tin. Roast for $1^3/_4$ hours, or until the chicken is golden, crisp, and cooked through. Halfway through cooking, pour a little water into the bottom of the roasting tin and keep topping this up as it evaporates.

5 Transfer the cooked chicken to a warmed serving plate. Add a little extra water to the cooking juices, if necessary, and boil the liquid, scraping all the roasting residue off the pan. When the gravy is reduced and flavoursome, check the seasoning and serve a little poured over the chicken.

NUTRITIONAL VALUES

ROAST TOMATO CHICKEN CREOLE

SERVES **6**

This Louisiana Creole dish is based on a rich, spicy tomato sauce that is cooked long and slow, then served over rice.

5 chicken breasts, boned and skinned

1 tbsp flour

1 tsp salt substitute (see page 12)

$1/4$ tsp dried thyme

$1/2$ tsp dried marjoram (oregano)

$1/2$ tsp dried basil

$1/2$ tsp paprika

$1/8$ tsp cayenne

$1/8$ tsp freshly ground black pepper

$1/8$ tsp white pepper

4 tbsp olive oil, divided

100 g onion, chopped

100 g green pepper, chopped

100 g celery, chopped

2 cloves garlic, finely chopped

750 ml chicken stock (see page 25)

600 g fresh tomatoes, deseeded and chopped

225 g can tomato sauce

1 tsp sugar

few drops Tabasco sauce

15 g fresh parsley, chopped

75 g spring onions, chopped

600 g cooked rice

1 Cut the chicken into bite-size cubes. Mix the flour and spices in a small bowl. Sprinkle the spices over the chicken, and toss the chicken so the cubes are evenly covered with spice. Heat 2 tbsp oil in a frying pan. Sauté the chicken until it is lightly browned and cooked through, about 10 minutes. Remove the chicken with a slotted spoon, and set aside.

2 Add the additional oil to the pan, if necessary. Sauté the onion, pepper, celer, and garlic for 5 minutes.

3 In a large saucepan, bring the chicken stock to the boil. Add the chicken, sautéed vegetables, tomatoes, tomato sauce, and sugar. Simmer, covered, for 45 minutes, stirring occasionally. Add Tabasco and salt to taste. Just before serving, stir in the parsley and spring onions. Spoon the Creole sauce over rice in bowls and serve.

NUTRITIONAL VALUES

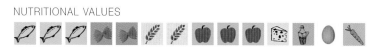

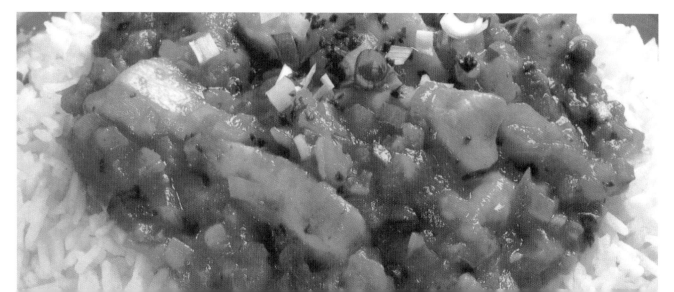

ARMENIAN-STYLE CHICKEN AND CHICKPEA STEW

SERVES **6**

The Armenians have a spicy condiment sold as Aintab Red Pepper in the West. Since it is difficult to find, two thin medium-hot red peppers have been substituted here.

4 threads saffron

125 ml hot water

10 cloves garlic, crushed

2 fresh thin medium-hot red peppers, deseeded and chopped

4 tbsp olive

1.3 kg chicken breasts and thighs, washed and dried

freshly ground black pepper

2 tbsp ground coriander

1 tsp dried marjoram (oregano)

2 x 400 g cans plum tomatoes, drained

480 ml water

600 g can chickpeas, drained

2 tbsp lemon juice

1   Soak the saffron in hot water for 10 minutes. Place the saffron and liquid, garlic and peppers in a blender or food processor. Process until finely chopped and set aside.

2   Heat the oil in a casserole over medium-hot heat. Season the chicken to taste, and sauté in batches until lightly browned. Remove to a plate and keep warm.

3   Reduce the heat and add the crushed garlic. Stir with a wooden spoon for 2 minutes, then add the ground coriander and marjoram (oregano). Stir for a further 2 minutes, then add the tomatoes. Break them up with the spoon while cooking for 3 minutes, then add the water. Add the chicken pieces and spoon the sauce over them. Bring to the boil, cover, and simmer over low heat for 20 minutes.

4   Add the chickpeas and continue to cook, covered, for a further 15 minutes. Remove the lid, stir in the lemon juice, and increase the heat. Boil for 5 minutes to reduce the sauce. Serve immediately.

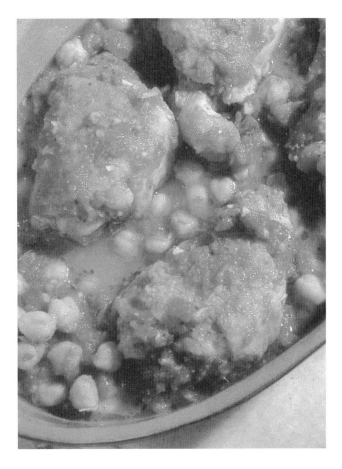

NUTRITIONAL VALUES

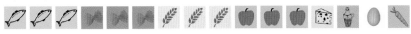

BACON HOTPOT WITH DELICIOUS DUMPLINGS

SERVES **4**

A delicious meal of bacon and vegetables with dumplings, ideal for cold wet days.

1 tbsp olive oil

450 g boneless ham, cubed

1 large onion, chopped

2 tbsp all-purpose flour

625 ml bacon, chicken (see page 25) or vegetable
stock (see page 24)

250 ml unsweetened apple juice

200 g carrots, sliced

200 g parsnips, cubed

400 g ratabaga or celery root, cubed

freshly ground black pepper

450 g brussels sprouts, halved if large

DUMPLINGS

125 g self-raising flour

1 tsp baking powder

250 g fresh whole-meal breadcrumbs

100 g rolled oats

2 tbsp fresh parsley, chopped

2 tsp fresh sage, chopped, or 1 tsp dried sage

4 spring onions, chopped

125 ml low-fat cream cheese

125 ml skimmed milk

1 Heat the oil, add the ham and brown the pieces lightly, then add the onion and continue cooking for about 10 minutes, or until the onion is softened. Stir in the flour and pour in the stock. Bring to the boil stirring, then pour in the apple juice.

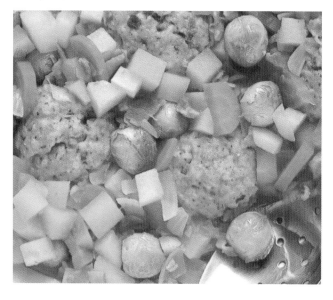

2 Add the carrots, parsnips and rutabaga or celery root with seasoning. Reduce the heat so the liquid is just simmering, cover and continue to cook gently for 30 minutes.

3 For the dumplings, mix the flour, baking powder, breadcrumbs, oatmeal and parsley with the sage and spring onions. Make a well in the middle of the mixture. Beat the cheese with the milk, then add it to the dry ingredients and mix together thoroughly.

4 Divide the mixture in half, then shape each half into four round dumplings. Add the sprouts to the hotpot and stir, then place the dumplings on top and cover tightly. If the dumplings are too high for the lid, tent foil over the top of the pan, tucking it around the rim to keep in the steam.

5 Simmer for 20 minutes, until the dumplings are risen and cooked through. Use a slotted spoon to transfer the dumplings to serving plats, then ladle the bacon and vegetable mixture beside them. Serve at once.

NUTRITIONAL VALUES

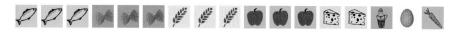

STUFFED BAKED POTATOES

SERVES **4**

A couple of ideas to serve up in a nice hot baked potato!

4 even-sized large potatoes

CHICKEN WITH SWEETCORN

225 g cooked chicken, chopped

1 green pepper, deseeded and chopped

4 tbsp sweetcorn, cooked

2 tbsp mayonnaise

2 tomatoes, skinned

freshly ground black
    pepper

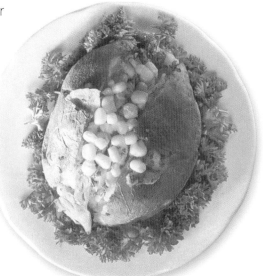

1   Wash and brush the potato skins. Prick with a fork.

2   Arrange on the oven shelves and bake for 45–60 minutes at 200°C/gas mark 6. Alternatively, boil the potatoes for 15 minutes, drain and then bake in the oven for 25–35 minutes, depending on size. Potatoes can also be baked in a microwave oven – one potato will take 5 minutes but four will need 20 minutes. Crisp in the oven if liked.

3   Cut the potato lengthwise and scoop out some of the potato, reserve, and mix with filling.

4   Fill the potatoes with fillings to suit individual tastes and reheat for a few minutes in the oven.

5   Potatoes can be prepared and stuffed and kept in the refrigerator until needed. Heat through before serving.

BAKED BEANS AND BACON

1 small can baked beans

4 slices streaky bacon

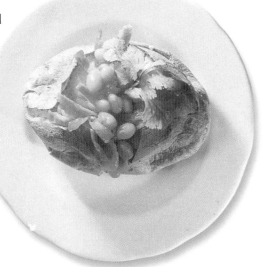

1   Mix the beans with the potato filling.

2   Grill the bacon until crisp. Break into small pieces.

3   Fill the potatoes with the bean mixture, arrange crispy bacon on top. Reheat.

NUTRITIONAL VALUES

SALAD OF FRENCH LENTILS AND GRILLED OR BARBECUED MUSHROOMS

SERVES **4**

A little marinating lets the flavours permeate the mushrooms and keeps them juicy during grilling or barbecuing. A grilled sausage served with the mushrooms turns this salad into a complete meal.

175 g French Puy lentils

3 bay leaves

750 ml water

3 large flat mushrooms or portobellos

5 cloves garlic, chopped

3 shallots, chopped

3–5 tbsp walnut oil

2–3 tbsp balsamic or sherry vinegar

salt substitute (see page 12) and freshly ground
    black pepper, to taste

2 tbsp each chopped fresh parsley, thyme, or
    savory

a handful of mixed salad greens

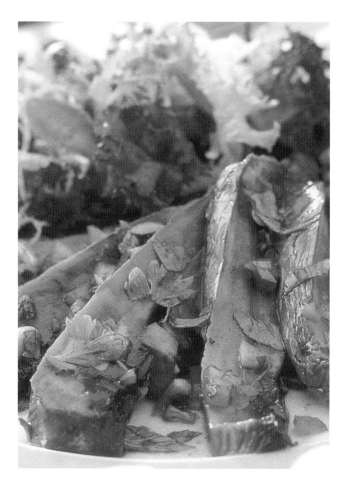

1 Combine the lentils with the bay leaves and water, and bring to the boil. Reduce the heat and simmer, covered, until the lentils are just tender, about 30–40 minutes. Do not let them fall apart. Drain well and discard the bay leaves.

2 Meanwhile, remove the stalks from the mushrooms. Sprinkle the top of the mushrooms with about half of the garlic, shallots, walnut oil, vinegar, salt substitute, pepper and herbs.

3 Heat the grill or barbecue, and cook the mushrooms, skin side down, letting the juices accumulate in their caps. When they are tender and cooked through, remove from the heat and slice.

4 Arrange a portion of lentils (they can be either warm or cool) on each plate. Toss the greens with a few spoonfuls of the remaining shallots, garlic, oil, vinegar, salt substitute, pepper and herbs, then arrange this on the plates next to the lentils. Arrange the mushrooms on each plate and sprinkle the remaining oil, vinegar, shallots, garlic and herbs over it all. Serve immediately.

NUTRITIONAL VALUES

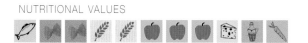

FEIJOADA

SERVES **4**

Feijoada, *a spicy stew of black beans and pork, is the ceremonial dish of Brazil. Traditionally it is made with various parts of the pig, such as snout, ears, tail and trotters. This hot Americanized version uses pork loin and linguica, a garlicky Portuguese sausage.*

350 g dried black beans, picked
    over and soaked overnight

4 tbsp olive oil

3 dried chillies de arbol, whole

8 cloves garlic, crushed

900 g pork loin, cubed

1 large onion, chopped

425 g can tomatoes, chopped

450 g linguica, cut into 5 mm
    slices

3 jalapeño chillies, deseeded,
    minced

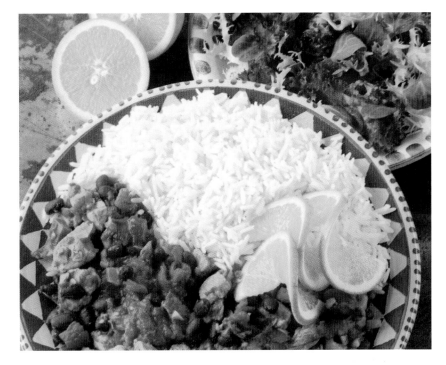

1 Drain the beans, put them in a stockpot and add enough water to cover 5 cm. Bring to the boil, reduce heat and simmer.

2 Heat 1 tablespoon of the oil in a small frying pan and sauté the chillies de arbol and half the crushed garlic for 1–2 minutes, until the garlic just starts to brown. Add to the beans. Heat another 1 tablespoon oil in a large frying pan and cook the pork until lightly browned. Add the pork to the beans. Heat the remaining oil in a frying pan and sauté the onion and remaining half of the crushed garlic for 5 minutes, then add to the beans.

3 Add the tomatoes and linguica to the beans. Return the stew to the boil, reduce heat and simmer. When beans have simmered for 1 hour, add the jalapeños. Continue simmering until the beans are tender, a total of 1½–2 hours.

NUTRITIONAL VALUES

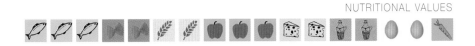

PORK PARCELS

SERVES **4**

These can be served in their foil so you get to open the parcels yorself, and can be garnished with sage leaves.

50 g long grain rice

175 g frozen peas, defrosted

100 g frozen sweetcorn, defrosted

1 onion, chopped

salt substitute (see page 12) and freshly ground
   black pepper

4 x 100 g pork fillets or tenderloin steaks

1 tsp French mustard

1 tsp fresh sage, chopped

4 tbsp cider

fresh sage leaves (optional), to garnish

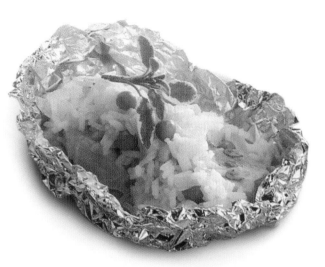

1 Place the rice in a saucepan of boiling water and cook for 10 minutes. Drain.

2 Mix the peas, sweetcorn, onion and rice together and season.

3 Place each of the pork steaks on a large sheet of aluminium foil. Spread with mustard and sprinkle with sage.

4 Place a quarter of the rice mix on each steak, add a spoonful of cider and fold over the foil to make four sealed parcels.

5 Bake in a preheated oven at 180°C/gas mark 4 for 45 minutes.

6 Serve either straight from the foil or unwrap and place on individual warmed plates and garnish with sage leaves.

NUTRITIONAL VALUES

JERKED BEEF KEBABS

SERVES **6**

The marinade for these kebabs is deeply flavoursome. Enjoy with a rice dish or baked potatoes and a crisp green salad.

3 tbsp olive oil

1 onion, roughly chopped

2 tbsp lemon juice

1½ tbsp dried thyme

1½ tbsp ground cinnamon

1½ tbsp sugar

1 tbsp chilli sauce

1½ tsp ground coriander

1½ tsp grated nutmeg

1 tsp salt substitute (see page 12)

1 tsp freshly ground black pepper

1 kg blade, sirloin, or rump steak, cut into 3 cm
   cubes

1 Put all the ingredients, except the steak, into a blender or food processor and blend until smooth. Pour into a large, shallow non-metallic dish.

2 Add the steak, stirring until well coated. Cover and leave to marinate for 2 hours or chilled for longer, stirring occasionally.

3 Thread the steak onto six flat metal skewers then, cook over medium-high heat for 6–8 minutes, turning occasionally, until cooked to your liking.

NUTRITIONAL VALUES

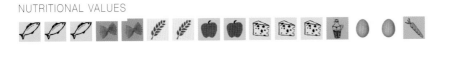

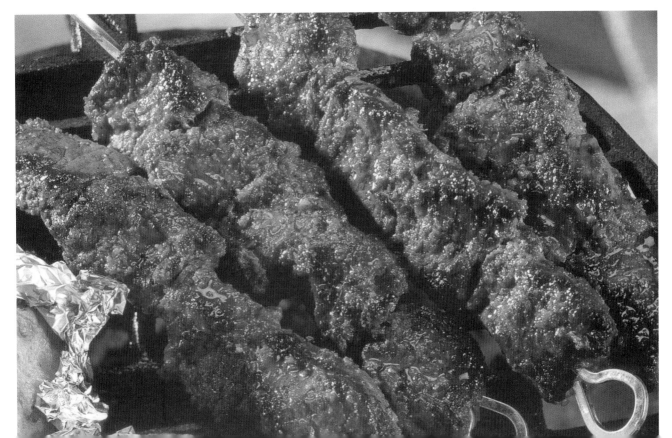

CALIFORNIA FIVE-WAY CHILLI

SERVES **6 – 8**

This variation of Cincinnati chilli uses Mexican ingredients that have become staples in California kitchens: chorizo sausage, black beans, coriander and a combination of unsweetened cocoa, cinnamon and cloves that are reminiscent of molé dishes. It is pleasantly spicy.

625 g ground beef

225 g chorizo sausage (not smoked)

1 onion, chopped

3 cloves garlic, crushed

2 tsp unsweetened cocoa

1 tsp cinnamon

1/4 tsp ground cloves

1 tsp ground cumin

1 tsp dried marjoram

2 tbsp chilli powder

1 tbsp hot or Mexican chilli powder

1 tbsp red wine vinegar

175 ml tomato purée

15 g fresh coriander, chopped

about 1 tsp salt substitute (see page 12)

450 g can black beans

350 g spaghetti, cooked

1 1/2 onions, chopped

225 g Cheddar cheese, grated

1 Brown the ground beef in a frying pan. Spoon off the excess fat, put the meat in a large saucepan and set aside. Brown the chorizo sausage in a frying pan. Drain off all but 1 tablespoon of the fat, and remove the sausage with a slotted spoon. Add the sausage to the saucepan. Reheat the fat and sauté the onion and garlic for 5 minutes. Add to the saucepan.

2 Add the cocoa and seasonings to the saucepan. Add the vinegar and tomato purée and 450 ml water. Bring the mixture to the boil, stirring well. Reduce heat and simmer for about 1 1/4 hours, adding water if necessary. Add the coriander and salt substitute to taste.

3 Traditionally, the beans are one of the five layers in five-way chilli, but if you wish to mix the beans into the chilli, do so now.

4 To serve, start with a layer of spaghetti, add the chilli, beans, chopped onion, and cheese.

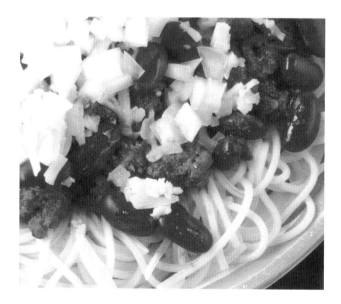

NUTRITIONAL VALUES

BEEF STEW WITH PASTA

SERVES **4**

This recipe is based on the Corsican Stufatu, but a few extra ingredients make it a hearty and filling dish.

FOR THE SAUCE

1 tbsp olive oil

1 large onion, peeled and chopped

2–3 cloves garlic, crushed

450 g stewing steak, trimmed and diced

2 tbsp seasoned flour

150 ml red wine

450 ml beef stock

salt substitute (see page 12) and freshly ground

black pepper

2 tbsp chopped fresh marjoram

4–6 baby carrots, trimmed

2 leeks, blanched and sliced

TO SERVE

275 g fresh fusilli

fresh Parmesan cheese, grated

fresh marjoram, chopped

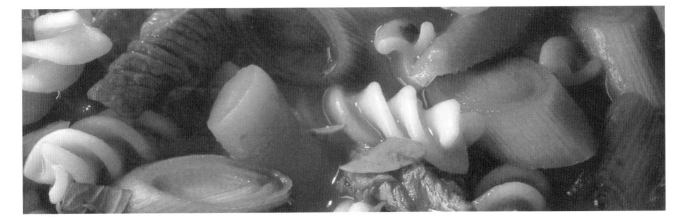

1   Preheat the oven to 180°C/gas mark 4, 10 minutes before cooking the stew. Heat the oil in a large pan and sauté the onion and garlic for 5 minutes or until softened but not browned.

2   Toss the meat in the seasoned flour, then add to the pan and brown, stirring frequently. Sprinkle in any remaining flour and cook for 2 minutes. Gradually stir in the wine and stock. Bring to the boil, stirring, then remove from the heat and stir in seasoning to taste; add the marjoram. Pour into a casserole dish, cover with a lid, and cook for 1$\frac{1}{2}$ hours.

3   Cut the carrots in half if large. Cook in boiling water for 3 minutes, drain and add to the stew with the leeks. Continue to cook for 30 minutes or until the meat is tender.

4   Meanwhile, cook the fusilli in plenty of boiling water for 1–2 minutes or until tender but firm to the bite. Drain and stir into the stew. Sprinkle with the grated Parmesan and marjoram and serve.

NUTRITIONAL VALUES

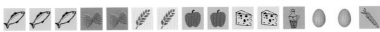

MIXED BEAN SALAD

SERVES **4**

This looks great served in the centre of tomato wedges, chicory leaves and thinly sliced cucumber.

100 g butter beans

100 g kidney beans

3 spring onions, washed

3 small peppers, yellow, green and red

8 slices salami

150 ml French dressing

2 tbsp parsley, chopped

GARNISH

2 heads chicory, sliced

2 tomatoes, cut into wedges

1/4 cucumber, thinly sliced

1 Soak the butter and kidney beans in separate bowls overnight. Cook in separate saucepans just covered with cold water, bring to the boil and simmer for 30–40 minutes, or until the beans are tender. Allow to cool.

2 Chop the spring onions. Deseed the peppers and cut into thin strips, dice the salami. Place all these ingredients in a bowl with the cold beans and French dressing, mix well. Add the chopped parsley and mix again.

3 Arrange the sliced chicory around a shallow bowl and surround with tomato wedges and cucumber. Pile the bean salad in the centre.

NUTRITIONAL VALUES

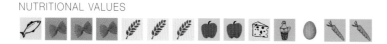

DESSERTS

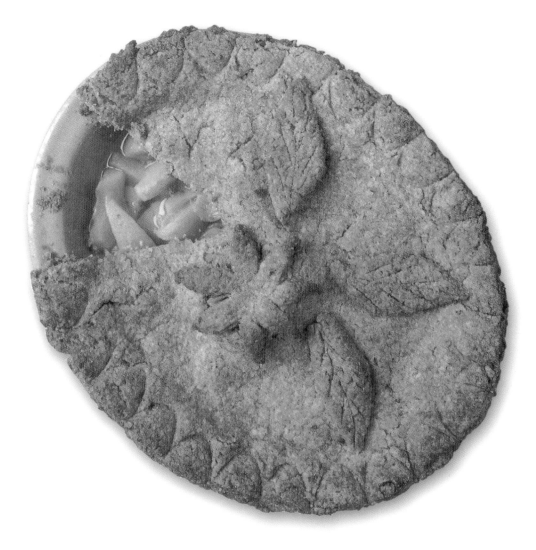

APRICOT TART

This tart is at its best when still warm from the oven.

450 g sweet or puff pastry

500 g fresh or canned apricots – which should be
   halves if possible

160 g icing sugar

9 tbsp apricot jam

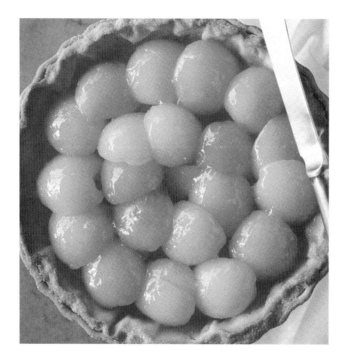

1 Line a flan ring with the pastry, prick all over and dust lightly with the icing sugar.

2 Halve the apricots and pit them, if fresh. Line the pastry case with the fruit, so that each piece slightly overlaps the one before it. Dust the remaining sugar over the fruit and bake the tart.

3 As the tart is cooking, melt the jam over gentle heat. Using a pastry brush, glaze the tart with the molten jam as soon as it is cooked.

NUTRITIONAL VALUES

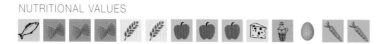

BANANA AND RHUBARB FOOL

SERVES **6**

Bananas and rhubarb are a wonderful combination of fruits for crumbles, pies and fools. Toss the banana slices in lime juice, which not only stops them browning but also brings out the flavour of the rhubarb.

450 g cooked rhubarb pieces, fresh or canned

3 large bananas, sliced

125 ml rhubarb juice or syrup

grated rind and juice of 1 lime

2 pieces preserved ginger, finely chopped

50 ml honey

225 g plain low-fat yoghurt

15 g wheat germ

1 Purée the rhubarb, banana, rhubarb juice, lime rind and juice in a blender or food processor. Turn into a bowl and add the ginger with honey to taste. Fold the yoghurt into the mixture with the wheat germ, then cover and chill for 1–2 hours. Serve decorated with a little extra wheat germ.

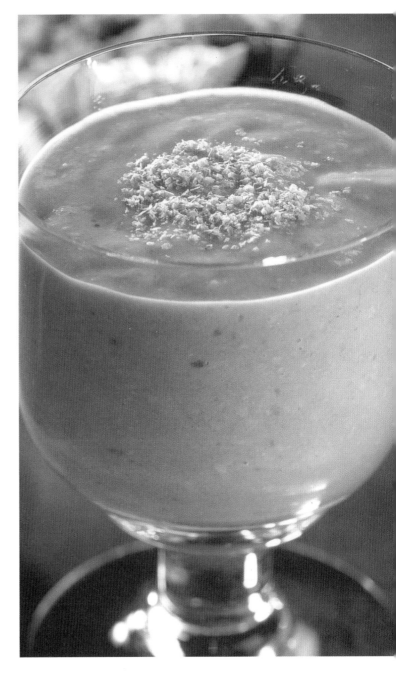

NUTRITIONAL VALUES

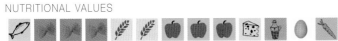

SUMMER PUDDING

SERVES **6**

This is a delightful way to celebrate the soft fruit harvest or to utilize a store of frozen currants and berries.

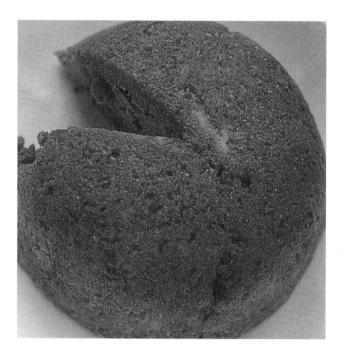

1 kg mixed soft fruits such as raspberries,
    gooseberries and blackcurrants
50 g light muscovado sugar, or to taste
3–4 tbsp water
about 8 slices wholemeal bread cut from a large
    loaf, crusts removed

DECORATION

scented geranium or other herb leaves (optional)

1 Prepare the fruit as required; hull raspberries, top and tail gooseberries, and strip blackcurrants from the stalks. Put the fruit into a large pan with the sugar and water and cook over a low heat until the sugar dissolves and the juices start to run. Cook gently until all the fruit is just tender – about 15 minutes.

2 Cut the bread slices to line a 900 ml bowl or basin. Fit the bread around the container so that there are no gaps.

3 Tip the fruit into the basin and cover the top with more bread slices so that the fruit is completely enclosed. Place a saucer or small plate over the container and press it down with a heavy weight.

4 Leave the pudding in the refrigerator for several hours or overnight. To unmould the pudding, run a knife blade between the basin and the bread lining, place a serving plate over the top, invert both pudding and plate, and shake sharply to release the pudding. Decorate with the herb leaves. Serve with fromage frais or crème fraîche if wished.

NUTRITIONAL VALUES

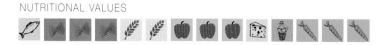

BAKED PASTA PUDDING

SERVES **4**

A nursery pudding which will probably become a firm favourite with the adults.

100 g dried tagliatelle

dash of sunflower oil

50 g butter

2 eggs

100 g granulated sugar

pinch of ground cinnamon

grated zest of 1 lemon

few drops vanilla essence

4 tbsp sultanas

sifted icing sugar, to decorate

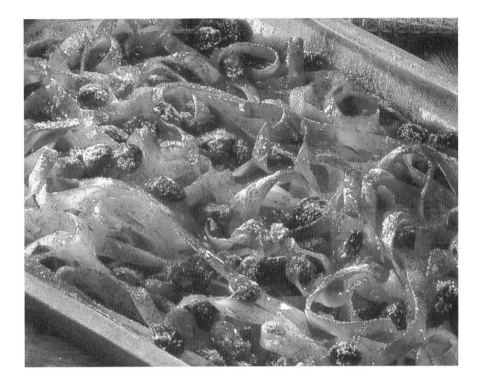

1 Preheat the oven to 190°C/gas mark 5. Bring a large saucepan of water to the boil and add the tagliatelle with a dash of sunflower oil. Cook for about 10 minutes, stirring occasionally, until tender. Drain and rinse under cold running water. Drain again and set aside.

2 Place the butter in a shallow ovenproof dish and melt in the oven for about 5 minutes. Remove from the oven and carefully swirl the melted butter around the sides of the dish. Set aside to cool slightly.

3 In a mixing bowl, whisk together the eggs and sugar until thick and frothy. Whisk in the cinnamon, lemon zest, vanilla essence and reserved melted butter. Stir in the sultanas and cooked tagliatelle until evenly coated in the egg mixture.

4 Transfer the pudding mixture to the prepared dish and distribute evenly. Bake for about 35–40 minutes, until the mixture has set and is crisp and golden. Allow to cool slightly. Serve warm, decorated with sifted icing sugar.

NUTRITIONAL VALUES

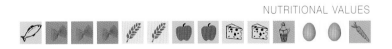

DRIED FRUIT COMPOTE

Any combination of fruits can be used and the poaching liquid can range from water to tea, fruit juice or wine. You can experiment with this. Serve with a dollop of yoghurt or sour cream to cut the natural sweetness.

215 g large pitted prunes

215 g dried no-soak apricots

215 g dried no-soak pears

100 g dried no-soak peaches

100 g dried no-soak apple rings

90 g raisins

4 tbsp honey or sugar (optional)

grated zest and juice of 1 lemon

grated zest and juice of 1 orange

4–6 whole cloves

1 cinnamon stick

1 tbsp black peppercorns (optional)

slivered blanched almonds, toasted, for garnish

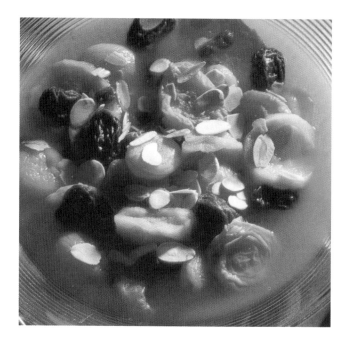

1   Into a large non-aluminum saucepan, place prunes, apricots, pears, peaches, apple rings, and raisins. Cover with 2 litres of water or enough to generously cover fruit.

2   Stir in honey or sugar to taste, if using, and add grated lemon and orange zests and juices, cloves, cinnamon stick and peppercorns, if using. Over high heat, bring to the boil. Cook, covered, over low heat, until fruit is plump and tender, 20 minutes.

3   With slotted spoon, remove cloves, cinnamon stick and peppercorns. Spoon fruit into a serving bowl and pour liquid over. Chill 3–4 hours or overnight. Sprinkle with toasted almonds for garnish and serve with low-fat yoghurt or low-fat sour cream.

NUTRITIONAL VALUES

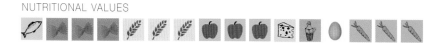

RHUBARB STREUSEL CAKE

MAKES 1 large cake

This may be served hots as a pudding, or cold as a cake. The crumb topping gives a delicious crunch in contrast to the rhubarb, which softens into the cake mix. Apples and gooseberries are good alternatives to the rhubarb.

STREUSEL TOPPING

90 g butter

120 g wholemeal flour

1/2 tsp baking powder

120 g demerera sugar

CAKE

120 g butter or unsaturated margarine

150 g brown sugar

2 large eggs, beaten

120 g wholemeal flour

1 tsp baking powder

1/2 tsp ground cinnamon

1 tbsp milk

175 g rhubarb pieces, in 5 cm lengths, fresh or canned

1 Preheat the oven to 175°C/gas mark 4, then line a 20 cm deep, round cake tin with baking parchment.

2 First prepare the topping. Blend the butter into the flour, baking powder and sugar until evenly distributed, then set aside. Cream the butter and sugar until pale and fluffy then gradually add the beaten egg. Mix together the flour, baking powder and cinnamon, then fold them into the mixture, adding the milk to give a soft dropping consistency.

3 Spoon the cake mixture into the prepared tin and roughly smooth the top. Arrange the rhubarb over the sponge then cover with the topping mixture, spreading it evenly.

4 Bake for 1 hour, or until a toothpick inserted into the cake comes out clean. Leave in the tin for 2–3 minutes, then remove the cake carefully, peel off the paper, and leave to cool completely on a wire rack.

NUTRITIONAL VALUES

APRICOT MUESLI BARS

These fruit muesli bars make a substantial snack or a light meal.

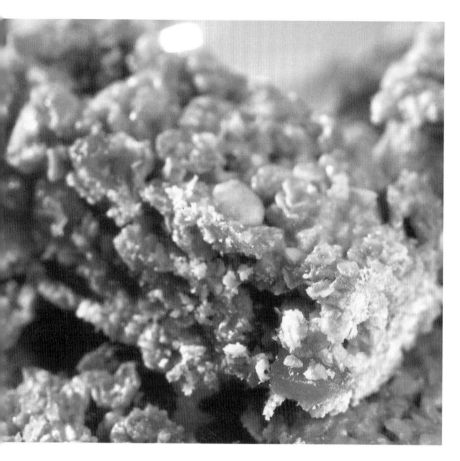

50 g unsaturated margarine

90 g honey

120 g muesli

60 g wholemeal flour

FILLING

150 g dried apricots, finely chopped

grated rind and juice of 1 orange

1 Preheat the oven to 190°C/gas mark 5 and lightly grease an 18 cm square cake tin.

2 Cook the apricots with the orange rind and juice, simmering slowly until all the orange juice has disappeared. Allow to cool until needed. Melt the margarine in a pan, add the honey and heat gently until melted into the margarine. Stir in the muesli and flour and mix well.

3 Press half the muesli mixture into the prepared cake tin then cover with a layer of apricots. Top with the remaining muesli mixture, pressing it down and smoothing the top with a metal spoon. Try to push any raisins into the mixture so they do not overcook.

4 Bake for 20–25 minutes, until lightly browned. Mark into bars and allow to cool in the tin. Cut through then cool completely on a wire rack. Store in an airtight container.

NUTRITIONAL VALUES

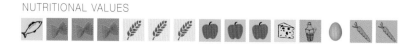

PRUNE AND WALNUT TART

SERVES **6**

Baked in a crisp pastry and made with cream for a special occasion. One mouthful of this tart conjures up images of prune country in southwestern France.

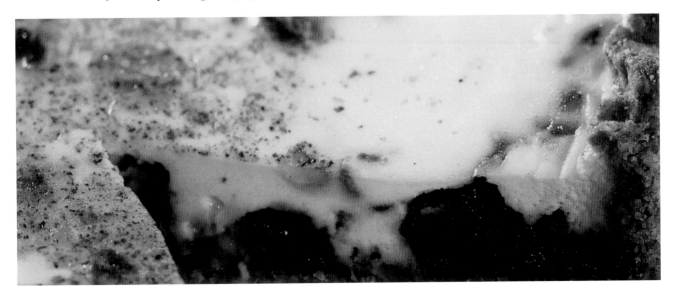

PASTRY

90 g butter

150 g fine wholemeal flour

1 tbsp light brown sugar

1 large egg, beaten

2 tbsp plum jam or apple jelly

120 g prunes, stoned, roughly chopped

300 ml ml milk

2 large eggs, beaten

1 tsp granulated sugar (optional)

freshly grated nutmeg

1 Prepare the pastry by blending the butter into the flour and sugar. Bind with the beaten egg then knead gently on a lightly floured surface. Cover the pastry with plastic wrap and chill in the refrigerator for 30 minutes.

2 Preheat the oven to 200°C/gas mark 6. Roll out the pastry to line a deep, 20 cm flan or cake tin, preferably loose-bottomed. Fill the pastry case with baking parchment and baking beans, then bake for 15 minutes. Remove the baking beans and parchment and continue cooking for a further 5 minutes, until the base is dry.

3 Reduce the oven heat to 175°C/gas mark 4. Spread the jam over the base of the pastry case then top with the prunes and walnuts. Beat the milk with the eggs and sugar, if used, then pour the custard into the pastry case and shred some nutmeg over the top. Bake for 40 minutes, or until the custard is lightly set. Leave to cool, then serve warm or cold.

NUTRITIONAL VALUES

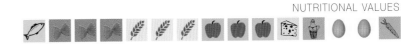

ORANGE AND BANANA MUFFINS

MAKES **six 4-in muffins**

A delicious recipe that makes six muffins; if more are needed just double the quantity.

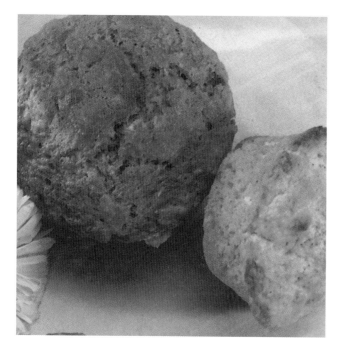

90 g plain wholemeal flour

60 g rolled oats

75 g unbleached plain flour

1 tbsp baking powder

75 g soft brown sugar

$^1/_2$ tsp salt substitute (see page 12)

3 tbsp wheat germ

1 tsp ground cinnamon

125 ml orange juice, freshly squeezed

1 size-3 egg, lightly beaten

2 bananas, mashed

2 tbsp grateed orange zest

60 g unsalted butter, melted

1   Preheat oven to 200°C/gas mark 6.

2   Grease six 7.5 cm deep bun tins.

3   In a large bowl, combine the dry ingredients. In a small bowl, combine all the remaining ingredients, mixing well. Add the liquid ingredients to the dry ones all at once and stir just until moistened. Spoon the mixture into the prepared tins, filling them $^2/_3$ full.

4   Bake for about 25 minutes, or until they are golden brown and a wooden toothpick inserted in the centre of a muffin comes out clean.

NUTRITIONAL VALUES

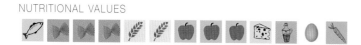

PEACHES AND PEARS PIE

SERVES **6**

A delicious nutty pastry which complements the peaches and pears beautifully!

450 g can peach slices in natural juice

4 ripe pears, peeled, cored and sliced

grated peel of 1 orange

PASTRY

125 g wholemeal flour

70 g unsaturated margarine

150 g chopped walnuts

grated peel and juice of 1
orange

4 tbsp artificial sweetener

1 Preheat the oven at 200°C/gas mark 6.

2 Mix the peaches and their juice with the pears in a pie dish or baking dish.

3 Place the flour in a bowl, then cut in the margarine. Stir in the walnuts, orange peel and artificial sweetener with enough orange juice to bind the mixture.

4 Roll out the nut pastry dough slightly larger than the top of the pie dish. Cut a strip and dampen the edge of the dish, then press the strip on the rim of the dish. Dampen the dough rim and lift the rest of the dough over. Seal the edges and use any trimmings to decorate the pie – cut out shapes or leaves and dampen them to keep them in place.

5 Brush with a little milk and bake for about 30 minutes, or until the pastry is cooked and browned. Serve piping hot.

NUTRITIONAL VALUES

CRANACHAN

SERVES **4**

A very creamy and nutty treat to end any delicious meal.

50 g flaked almonds

50 g medium oatmeal

300 ml low-fat whipping cream

4 tbsp honey, to taste

4 tbsp whisky

1 tbsp lemon juice

raspberries

1 Toast the almonds and oatmeal.

2 Whip the low-fat cream in a bowl, and stir in the honey and whisky. Fold in the almonds and oatmeal, and finally, the lemon juice. Serve in tall glasses garnished with raspberries.

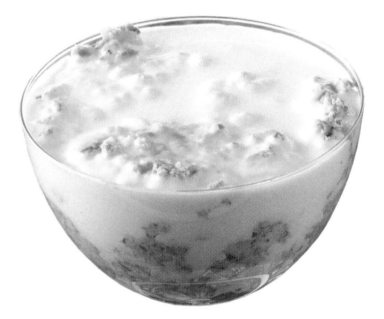

NUTRITIONAL VALUES

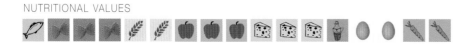

APPLE AND OATMEAL CAKE

SERVES **4**

This is best served with low-fat crème fraîche while it is still warm.

675 g cooking (tart) apples, peeled and sliced

4 tbsp brown sugar

1 tsp cinnamon

50 g raisins

FOR THE OATMEAL PASTRY

100 g unsalted butter

1 heaped tbsp brown sugar

2 tbsp clear honey

zest of 1 lemon

275 g medium oatmeal

2 eggs, beaten

1 glass whisky

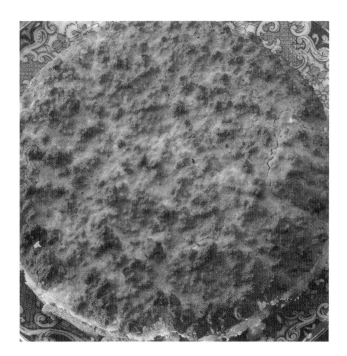

1   Preheat the oven 190°C/gas mark 5. Cook the apples, sugar and cinnamon in a saucepan until the apples form a pulp. Then add the raisins and cool.

2   Melt the butter, sugar, and honey in another saucepan. In a bowl, mix the oatmeal and lemon zest together, then pour into the honey mixture. Add the eggs and whiskey and mix well.

3   Divide the oatmeal mixture into three. Put one layer of the oatmeal on the bottom of a greased cake tin. Cover with half the apple mixture. Top this with another layer of oatmeal. Then add the final apple layer, then finish off with the oatmeal.

4   Bake for half an hour. Serve warm with low-fat crème fraîche.

NUTRITIONAL VALUES

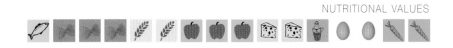

SLICED EXOTIC FRUITS WITH DATES

SERVES **6**

Almost any seasonal fruits are delicious sliced or cut up together in their natural juices or with a fruit purée. This is not a traditional fruit salad, but a selection of exotic fruits, sliced and served together.

1 Ogen melon, deseeded and sliced in thin
   wedges and peeled

3 sweet seedless oranges, peeled and segmented,
   juice reserved

1 mango, peeled and thinly sliced

24 fresh lychees, peeled, or 425 g can lychees in
   their own juice

12 Medjool dates, cut in half lengthwise and stoned

1 pomegranate, cut in half, seeds reserved
   (optional)

fresh mint leaves for garnish

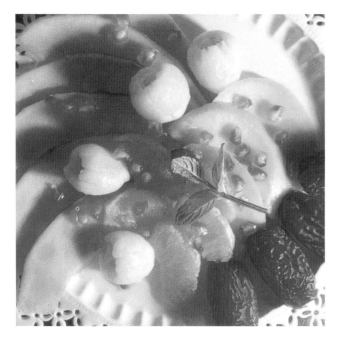

1 Arrange slices of melon on each of 6 individual plates in a fan shape. Arrange peeled orange segments and mango slices in an attractive pattern over the melon slices.

2 Evenly distribute fresh or canned lychees over fruit and sprinkle on some reserved juices from all fruits.

3 Arrange 4 date halves on each plate and sprinkle over the pomegranate seeds, if using. Garnish with fresh mint leaves and serve.

NUTRITIONAL VALUES

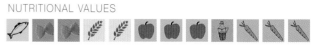

MUESLI COOKIES

MAKES **20**

These sweet cookies are very quick to make, but they must be chilled before baking or they will spread too much in the oven. The honey binds the mixture together; no egg is used. Work the dough well to produce light cookies.

120 g butter or unsaturated margarine

120 g light brown sugar

60 g honey

175 g muesli

120 g wholemeal flour

1 Cream the butter and sugar until pale and fluffy then add the honey and beat thoroughly again. Work in the muesli and flour to give a stiff dough which is only slightly sticky, then turn out on to a lightly floured surface and knead firmly until the dough is easily manageable.

2 Form into a sausage shape, about 30 cm long, then cover in plastic wrap and chill in the refrigerator for at least 30 minutes.

3 Preheat the oven to 175°C/gas mark 4 and lightly grease 2 baking sheets. Cut the cookie dough into 20 pieces, form into balls then flatten slightly and place on the prepared baking sheets. Bake for 12–15 minutes, until firm enough to transfer to a wire rack to cool completely.

4 Store in an airtight container.

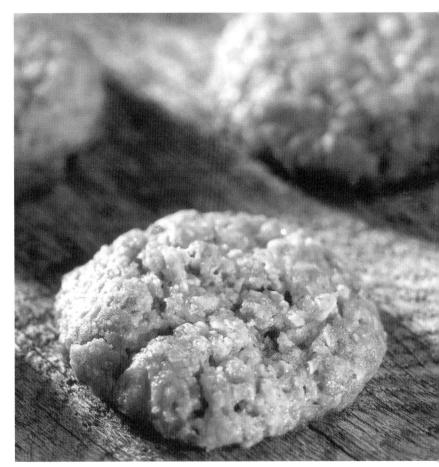

NUTRITIONAL VALUES

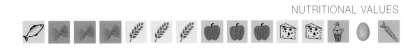

INDEX

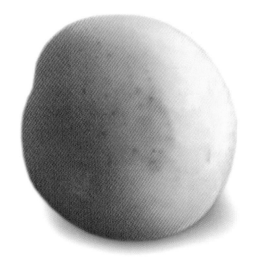